To the Faculty & students of Seton Hall University

Best wishes from a grateful alumnus!

Fred Buechel, MD '67

Principles of Human Joint Replacement

Frederick F. Buechel and Michael J. Pappas

Principles of Human Joint Replacement

Design and Clinical Application

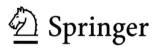 Springer

Authors

Prof. Frederick F. Buechel
UMDNJ
South Mountain Orthopaedics
61 First Street
South Orange
NJ 07079
USA
E-mail: buechelaakffb@yahoo.com

Prof. Michael J. Pappas
NJIT
8650 South Ocean Drive
Jensen Beach
FL 34957
USA
E-mail: mjpappas32@comcast.net

RD
686
.B885
2011

ISBN 978-3-642-23010-3   e-ISBN 978-3-642-23011-0

DOI 10.1007/978-3-642-23011-0

Library of Congress Control Number: 2011936700

Typeset & Cover Design: Scientific Publishing Services Pvt. Ltd., Chennai, India.

Printed on acid-free paper

9 8 7 6 5 4 3 2 1

springer.com

Preface

This book is written for the users and designers of joint replacements. It is an attempt to convey to the reader the knowledge accumulated by the authors during their thirty five year effort on the development of replacement devices for the lower limb for the purpose in aiding the reader in their design and evaluation of joint replacement devices.

Users include both the orthopaedic surgeons that implant such devices and patients who actually use the devices. The evaluation of such devices is far from simple and information provided by the manufacturer is usually self serving and often incomplete and inaccurate. There is relatively little information on long term experience with specific devices since most devices are abandoned before long term results are available. Thus, users should educate themselves sufficiently to allow independent evaluation of candidate devices in order to choose the best device available for the treatment of the pathology involved. This book provides information needed for such evaluation.

Patients should educate themselves on joint replacement since the selection of a device for use by a surgeon is often compromised by what is best for the surgeon. The selection of a device may be more dependent on the surgeons familiarity with the surgical procedure used to implant the device they select rather than the expected performance of the device. Further, many surgeons, particularly very successful surgeons, are provided with funding by a manufacturer for their collaboration and use of the manufacturers devices.

The history of joint replacement includes many triumphs and disasters. The triumphs are the result of clever individuals attempting to solve important human problems. The disasters are usually the result of the ignorance, or lack of application, of engineering and medical principles to the solution of complex problems. Designers of joint replacements should be familiar with past successes and failures so as to learn the lessons provided by them so as to apply successful features and not to repeat the errors of the past. Designers must also be capable of applying appropriate engineering, scientific and medical principles to the design, or redesign, of joint replacement so as to maximize their performance and minimize their risk. A primary purpose of this book is to provide and describe this history and such principles.

The first two chapters describe the engineering, scientific and medical principles needed for replacement joint evaluation. One must understand the nature and performance of the materials involved and their characteristics in vivo, i.e. the response of the body to implant materials. It is also essential to understand the response of the implants to applied loading and motion, particularly in the hostile physiological environment. The third chapter describes the design methodology now required for joint replacement in the USA and EU countries. The remaining chapters provide a history of joint replacement, an evaluation of earlier and current devices and description of the design rationale for some of the authors devices with which the authors are, of course, quite familiar.

Acknowledgements

The authors are grateful to Vincent J. Brier and Paul A. Witte for their work on the illustrations in this book and to Jared D. Pappas and Mark C. Buechel for their help in locating needed references and photographs and in proof reading and constructive comment on the text and figures.

Contents

Chapter 1
Properties of Materials Used in Orthopaedic Implant Systems

Abstract. This chapter describes the mechanical, physical, corrossive and biocompatability properties of materials used in orthopaedics. Titanium and Co-Cr-Mo alloys are used, almost exclusicely, for metalic implants. Of these the titanium alloy seems best suited for orthopaedic use due to its superior biocompatability, light weight, and low stiffnes and cost. Its poor abrasion esistance, however, makes the use of a hard coating, such as TiN ceramic necessary to produce a clearly superior metallic implant component. Aluminum alloys and stainless steels are used in instruments. Aluminum is used where low weight and low cost are important and great strength and abrasion resistance are not needed. Stainless steels of various types are employed in instruments. Austenitic 300 series is used where good corrosion resistance and strength are important but abrasion resistance is not. The 400 series steels are used where abrasion resistance is important such as in cutting tools and guides and some corrosion resistance can be sacrificed. The precipitation hardening steels are used where improved corrosion resisance is needed but at the sacricice of hardness and strength compared to the 400 series. UHMWPe is exclusively used for implant bearings with an highly cross-linked version commonly used for hip replacement bearings due to its apparent greatly improved wear resistance. The increased stiffness and brittlenes of the irradiation, however, makes the use if such materials in incongruent knees devices, questionable. Acetal and other engineering plastics are used for many instrument applications.

1.1 Introduction

An understanding of the properties of materials used in orthopedic implants and instruments is essential in the design and evaluation of such devices. Such understanding involves knowledge of mechanical and corrosion properties, and most importantly the biological reaction to such materials.

Mechanical properties involve an understanding of the concepts of stress and strain, stiffness, hardness, yielding, fracture and fatigue resistance. Corrosion involves an understanding of surface chemical properties and chemical reactions with the environment surrounding the orthopaedic devices. Biological interaction involves the reaction of the body to the release of toxic substances resulting from corrosion and wear in both the short and long term.

The science associated with material behavior in the physiological environment is very complex and not completely understood. This chapter, therefore, presents a rather simplified view of the concepts involved. A more complete understanding may be obtained from the references cited.

1.2 Mechanical Properties [1]

1.2.1 Stress and Strain

1.2.1.1 Stress

If a tensile load 'P' is applied to a specimen with an original cross section 'A' the resulting average tensile "stress", σ, is the value P/A. Values of such stress are always in terms of force per unit area such as PASCALS (Newtons/square meter). In most engineering applications the values are given in MPa or mega PASCALS, and will be used here exclusively.

1.2.1.2 Strain

The unit elongation, e, in the region of the minimum cross section is referred to as the "strain".

1.2.1.3 Stress – Strain Diagram

If one plots the stress vs. the stain for a tension test, for many metals, one obtains a "stress – strain diagram" as shown in Fig. 1.1.

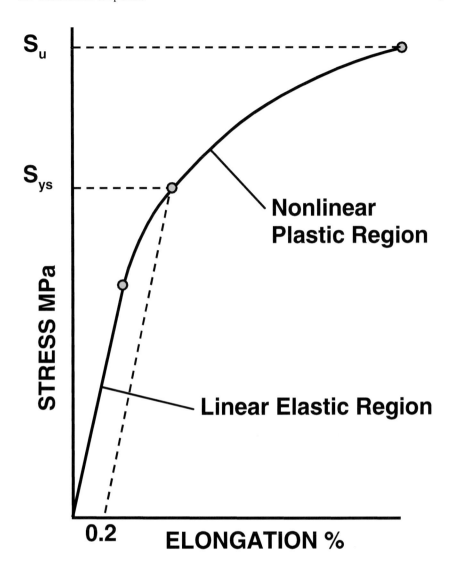

Fig. 1.1 Typical Stress – Strain Diagram for Many Metals.

Several important material characteristics may be obtained from such a diagram. These are:

1.2.1.4 Young's Modulus

This property is the value of σ/e in the "linear" region of the stress - strain curve. Its symbol is usually "E" and it represents the stiffness of the material. Since the units of strain is length vs. length (non-dimensional) the units of Young's Modulus, E, are the same as those of stress, σ.

1.2.1.5 Yield Point and Yield Strength

Most steels, and a few other metals, have a Stress – Strain Diagram of the form illustrated in Fig. 1.2.

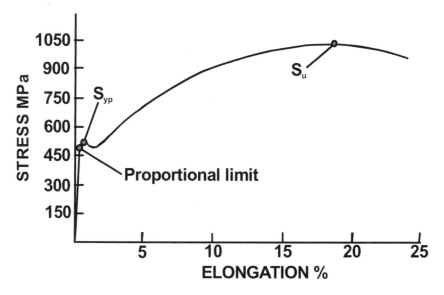

Fig. 1.2 Typical Stress – Strain Diagram for Steels.

Here, as may be seen, yielding occurs at an easily recognized stress. This value of stress is known as the "Yield Point", S_{yp}. Below this value of stress the test sample would return to its original shape and length. Above this value permanent deformation occurs.

For most metals used in orthopaedics, however, there is no such clearly defined yield point as may be seen from Fig. 1.1. Thus, one uses an arbitrary definition at which yielding occurs. Such a value is called the "Yield Strength" S_{ys}. Usually this is taken at the stress at which a permanent increase in the unit length of the test specimen test region of 0.20% has occurred.

The region of the stress strain diagram below the yield point or strength is called the "elastic" region and above the yield point or yield strength is called the "plastic" region.

1.2.1.6 Ultimate Strength

The highest value of stress on the stress strain diagram is the "Ultimate Stress" S_u. Normally the cross sectional area of the sample will be reduced by both the elastic and plastic deformation of the test. It should be noted that the original cross sectional area of the sample is used to compute the stress and not the reduced cross section resulting from elongation of the sample.

1.2.1.7 Poisson's Ratio

During tensile testing the elastic section of the specimen will become narrower and thinner in proportion to the original width and thickness of the region. The ratio of the dimensional reduction to the elongation of the region is called "Poisson's Ratio" and is usually symbolized by μ.

1.2.2 Hardness

Hardness is measured as the resistance to penetration by a specifically defined penetrator. The values are expressed in terms of numbers determined by a machine applying a specified load with a specified penetrator. For example the Rockwell hardness value scales ranging from A through G are used primarily for metals. The Vickers machine is used to test hardness of extremely hard metals and ceramics and the values measured are given by Vickers numbers. The scales are such that the greater the hardness number the harder the material.

1.2.3 Fatigue Resistance

The values obtained from a tensile test may be used for the stress analysis of a part under static loading. Under fluctuating loads, however, additional fatigue properties are needed to provide information on how designs may behave under such loading.

1.2.3.1 The SN Diagram

Most fractures are the result of a fluctuating load, well below the static failure stresses. Such fluctuating stresses result in "Fatigue" failure. A measure of materials ability to withstand repeated fluctuating stress is its "fatigue strength". Such values usually are determined by testing a carefully prepared, polished, circular beam specimen in a rotating test which subjects the outside surface of the beam to equal compressive and tensile stresses, the most damaging combination. A series of tests starts at stress values just below the yield strength of the material, where failure will occur relatively quickly. The stress for each subsequent test is incrementally reduced until failure does not occur. Plotted this data results in what is referred to as an "SN" curve as shown in Fig. 1.3.

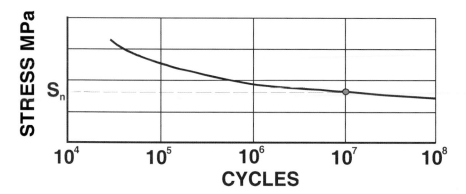

Fig. 1.3 Typical SN Curve for Many Metals.

The stress value, at which a sample fractures after a given number of cycles, usually 10^6 cycles, is the called fatigue strength S_n.

For most steels, however, failure will not occur below a certain stress even as the number of cycles of the test increase substantially beyond 10^6 cycles as illustrated in Fig. 1.4.

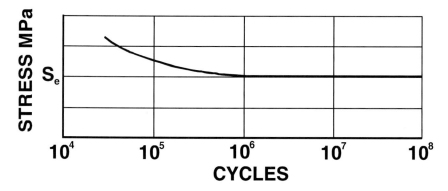

Fig. 1.4 Typical SN Curve for most Steels.

For such materials one refers to an "Endurance Limit" with the symbol S_e. This value should not be confused with fatigue strength where fatigue failure can occur after 10^6 cycles at stress values below the fatigue strength.

1.3 Corrosion Resistance

1.3.1 Metallic Corrosion

Metallic corrosion is primarily an electrochemical process that is dependent on electromotive potential, pH values and the environmental media. Even noble metals such as platinum and gold experience some dissolution and release of ions and formation of compounds. For noble metals, however, the degree of dissolution in almost all media is, fortunately, so small as to be essentially undetectable.

In a given media an electromotive potential below a certain value will produce "immunity" from corrosion. Above this value the level of pH determines if the metal will corrode or become "passive" by formation of a film on its surface. This film results from a chemical reaction with the media. [2]

For all metals used in orthopaedic implants today overall corrosion is so minor that it is not often readily observable. Observable corrosion in implants usually occurs locally in cracks, junctions between assembled parts, the inhomogineity of parts, or as a result of micro motion or stress.

Since instruments do not require as high a corrosion resistance as implants less corrosion resistant materials may be used to obtain advantages of cost, light weight and increased strength at the expense of reduced corrosion resistance. For such materials, particularly, aluminum and hardenable steel alloys overall corrosion can be a problem. To some extent acceptable levels of corrosion resistance for instruments using such metals may, however, be obtained by surface treatment after fabrication.

1.3.1.1 Galvanic Corrosion

This form of corrosion occurs generally at an area of contact of two materials with different electromotive potential in a conductive media. The contact between the metals of different electromotive potential creates an electromotive force. The presence of a conductive fluid essentially closes the circuit producing an electric current and thus, a flow of electrons much like in a battery. The metal to which the electrons flow is called the "cathode" and the metal from which the electrons flow the "anode".

All corrosion occurs at the anode unless the anode is made passive, which is not usually the case with most metal combinations. The cathode is always made immune.

1.3.1.2 Crevice Corrosion

A crevice usually occurs between mating parts. Corrosion can occur even with parts of identical material. Scratches, pits, machining marks or cracks can also provide conditions for such corrosion to occur. Differing immersion media conditions at the tip and mouth of the crevice possibly produce an ion concentration difference along the crevice producing galvanic "type" corrosion with anodic conditions in the crevice while the metal adjacent to the mouth acts as a cathode.

In the case of mating parts even minor differences in material resulting from batch to batch, heat treatment, and manufacturing process differences can accelerate crevice corrosion. Further, such corrosion often acts in concert with fretting from micro motion and fluctuating stress.

1.3.1.3 Stress Corrosion

Stress increases the energy in material under stress. This additional energy makes the metal more susceptible to corrosion. For most metals under static conditions it is of little importance. Static conditions are normally only the result of assembly forces. Applied, physiological loads are, however, generally fluctuating. Implant metals are generally corrosion resistant enough such that any additional corrosion due to constant stress is not significant. The same is true of most instruments since they spend relatively little time in a corrosive environment. The added effect of stress on corrosion becomes important where it is combined with galvanic and/or crevice corrosion.

1.3.1.4 Corrosion Fatigue

Fatigue due to fluctuating loading generally starts at some surface, or near a surface defect such as a scratch, pit, machining mark or metallic grain boundary (refer to Section 1.3.1.6 for more detail). At such points the combination of high stress due to stress concentration effects, crevice corrosion and stress corrosion greatly accelerates both corrosion and crack propagation substantially reducing fatigue strength and part life.

Little is known quantitatively about the effect of fatigue and strength as a result of such corrosion. It is of great importance, therefore to use the most corrosion resistant materials available in parts where corrosion fatigue is expected. Further, any fatigue testing of parts should be done in a medium simulating the body fluids to which the part is to be exposed.

1.3.1.5 Fretting Corrosion

Micro motion between assembled parts will typically produce wear debris, which due to its extremely large surface area per unit volume is much more susceptible to corrosive attack than the bulk material. This additional corrosion acts in concert with crevice corrosion to add to the tendency of corrosive products to increase wear by roughening the surfaces involved. This micro motion wear tends to disrupt any passive film or its development further increasing wear. Further, the stresses in the connecting parts will also accelerate wear.

Such wear can release significant amounts of toxic material. Thus, great care should be taken to avoid micro motion in implant assemblies or to avoid such assemblies altogether where possible.

1.3.1.6 Intergranular Corrosion

Almost all metal alloys are not homogeneous. Although when molten the alloying elements may be wholly soluble in the main metal and therefore, one would have a homogeneous molten metal. When the metal cools and solidifies, however, typically more than one form of metal crystal is formed. Often the one form will exist within the crystal and another at the boundary between crystals. In effect then one has within a metal two different metals providing potential for a galvanic type corrosion Thus, corrosion can begin at the boundary and if the boundary phase is anodic it can corrode producing a crevice thus further accelerating corrosion. Such a situation is particularly acute in castings.

To minimize such corrosion it is important to, not only use alloys with the best corrosion resistance available but to carefully select and control casting, heat treating processes and surface treatments.

1.3.2 Corrosion of Polymers

Since polymers are not conductive they are not subject to the effect of galvanic type corrosion. Rather, they are degraded by absorption from the media and dissolution in the media. UHMWPe is, for example, subject to oxidation in body fluids. Details of corrosion in polymers are generally poorly understood but it consists primarily of the effect of chemical reaction, absorption and leaching. The principal corrosion form in plastics affecting orthopaedic implants is "Stress Corrosion Cracking" and corrosion of fine wear particles.

1.3.2.1 Stress Corrosion Cracking

One similarity with metals is that corrosion in plastics is also accelerated by stress. Polymers that are normally quite resistant to a media may be readily attacked when under stress.

This is particularly true in crevices possibly due to differences in pH, ions and compounds in and outside the crevice. More likely such corrosion is due to the greatly magnified stress at the tip of the crack. This may be seen since accelerated corrosion of plastics under stress is characterized by the development and propagation of cracks perhaps leading to fracture. Fluctuating loading probably accelerate such corrosion. The effect is somewhat related to fatigue effects and the two effects probably work in tandem. Such cracking is illustrated in Fig. 1.5.

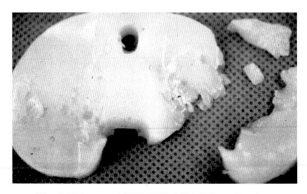

Fig. 1.5 Fractured UHMWPe Tibial Knee Bearing.

1.3.3 Corrosion of Ceramics

Most ceramics are generally almost immune to corrosion in body fluids. The strong ionic and covalent bonds of typical ceramics leave very little free chemical energy to aid corrosion [3]. Some Intergranular corrosion can occur in Aluminum Oxide ceramics due to impurities; however, such minor corrosion and its effects are generally imperceptible.

There are, of course, exceptions. In the 1980's yttria-stabilized tetragonal zirconia femoral heads were introduced due to their superior resistance to crack propagation, flexural strength and impact resistance. Unfortunately, the tetragonal phase is only metastable and can be transformed to a stable monoclinic by stress. In a study of 47 such heads, implanted from 2 through 10 years, Fernandez-Fairen et al [4] found a significant degradation of the heads due to reductions in fracture toughness. They also found increases in surface roughness and wear in the regions of the heads transformed to the monoclinic phase compared to the regions of the head where the tetragonal phase was retained.

1.4 Biological Response to Implants

Depending upon the location and application of implants and endoprostheses, various tissue and immunological responses have been identified. These responses generally include: foreign body encapsulation, tissue ingrowth or ongrowth, immunological sensitivity to materials and wear products and long-term function or failure of the implant.

1.4.1 Foreign Body Encapsulation

The human body tends to "wall off" or encapsulate any foreign body that comes in contact with subcutaneous or deeper tissues. In non-biocompatible foreign bodies, such as wooden splinters or the tip of a lead pencil, a series of inflammatory white blood cells surround the foreign bodies and cause tissue necrosis releasing cyto-toxic enzymes while trying to engulf the wood or lead, which are contaminated by bacteria that leads to infection. Fibrous tissue surrounds the "foreign bodies" which usually are "rejected" in a process of abscess formation that requires removal of the "foreign body" and the infected tissue to allow healing of the area.

In biocompatible foreign bodies, such as breast implants and artificial joints, the immune response is mild or non-reactive with the exception of "encapsulation" by fibrous tissue. The degree of cellular response to the foreign "implants" is variable and probably under genetic regulation of the host. When an "over-response" of fibrous encapsulation occurs, a hardness will be felt to the tissue surrounding breast implants and stiffness may be present in joint replacements that limit range of motion.

1.4.2 Tissue Ingrowth or Ongrowth

The surface characteristics of implants such as mechanical joint replacements can be altered to allow direct bone osseointegration for biological fixation. Such surfaces use microspheres or fiber-mesh bonded to the substrate metal and has a pore-size between 100 and 500 microns with a porosity of about 30% to allow tissue ingrowth for direct skeletal attachment. The ingrowth tissue is a mixture of fibrous tissue and bone. Usually, the more "biocompatible" the implant material, the more bone tissue ingrowth occurs.

Smooth implant surfaces usually allow tissue ongrowth, which may also be fibrous tissue or bone. Some materials, such as titanium, favor bone ongrowth, while plastics such as ultra-high molecular weight (UHMWPe) polyethylene or silicone and cobalt alloys favor fibrous tissue ongrowth.

1.4.3 Immunological Sensitivity to Material and Wear Products

Some patients are genetically predisposed to have allergies to certain implant materials such as nickel, cobalt or chromium. Some are allergic to bone cement (methyl methacrylate) used to fix implants to bone. Other patients develop sensitivity to these materials over time, when small diameter (often submicron in size) wear particles become phagocytized by white blood cells and stimulate an aggressive immune response that can cause loosening, pain or granuloma (walled-off sterile abscess) formation leading to implant failure.

1.4.4 Long Term Function or Failure of the Implant

Successful implant survival depends upon the body's tissue reaction to this "foreign body". In the best of circumstances, the implant or joint replacement will remain firmly attached and allow near-normal function for at least 10 years before wear or loosening start to occur. Superior joint replacement designs remain well-fixed to bone and continue to function for well-over 20 years before wear or fixation failure occurs. Unloaded implants with fibrous capsule stabilization, such as breast implants, can have lifetime function.

Infection or allergic sensitization over time are potential failure mechanisms that can occur during the lifespan of any implant. Such failures require implant removal and tissue stabilization. Subsequent reimplantation is possible using hypo allergenic materials to avoid recurrence.

1.5   Orthopaedic Materials

Almost all orthopaedic implant materials are conventional commercial materials, on occasion, modified for medical use. Most were developed more than a half century ago. There are, of course, exceptions such as biodegradable materials but such materials represent a very small fraction of those used in orthopaedic implants. Three materials, cobalt alloys such as Vitallium, titanium alloys such a Ti-4Al-6Va and UHMWPe are used in the overwhelming majority of orthopaedic implants.

1.5.1   Metals

1.5.1.1   Titanium

a) Introduction
The chemical element Titanium having the symbol Ti and an atomic number of 22 was discovered in England in 1791 and named for the Titans of Greek mythology. Its metallic forms are strong, light and extremely corrosion resistant. It is a metal of the "space age" [5].

Titanium compounds have been in wide use for some time. Titanium dioxide is used for white paint pigments and accounts for about 95% of the total use of the titanium element. But the use of the metal had been limited due to its high cost.

Titanium always occurs naturally in compound form with other elements. It is the ninth most abundant element in the earth's crust and the seventh most abundant metal. Its cost is primarily due to the difficulties of reducing the ore to metal. It is an extremely reactive metal and will burn in oxygen and nitrogen at its melting temperatures. Pure metallic titanium was first obtained in 1910 by M.A. Hunter. The cost of such extraction was such that it was not used outside the laboratory until an improved process was developed in 1932 by W.J. Krull.

The Soviet Union pioneered the use of Titanium alloys in submarine applications in the 1950's and 60's when they constructed two classes of submarines of such alloys. Russia today is the leading producer of titanium metals accounting for about 30% of world production. The United States pioneered the use of titanium alloys in military aircraft applications. It considered the material of strategic importance and the United States maintained a large stockpile until 2005.

The relatively high cost of the reduction of metallic titanium and the fabrication of titanium products had limited the applicability of its superior properties to a large number of non-military applications. In the last decade substantial advances have been made to reduce these costs. The recent FFC Cambridge process greatly decreases the cost of reduction. Improvements in cutting tools, lubricants and coolants have made the machining of Titanium alloys routine. Methods of casting titanium have been reduced to very successful commercial use. The majority of golf club drivers today are made of investment cast titanium alloy.

Titanium castings are often made by the investment casting process where metal molds produce wax parts around which a ceramic mold is created from a ceramic slurry. The wax is then melted and removed to create a ceramic mold into which the molten titanium is poured in a controlled atmosphere. Even with atmospheric controls, however, a thick, hard and brittle oxide case forms on the surface of the part. This case must then be removed by chemical milling. Still production casting processes have advanced to the point where titanium casting can be made economically at cost similar to cast cobalt alloys.

b) Physical Properties
Titanium occurs naturally in five stable isotopes [48]Ti being the most abundant and the one used in metallic form. At room temperature pure titanium has a hexagonal crystal form, its alpha phase. It changes to body centered cubic, its beta phase, at temperatures above 810° C. Alloying can change the phase transformation temperature and the rate of transformation. Thus, the high strength, heat treatable alloys are generally multiphase alloys.

The ASTM recognizes 31 grades of titanium metal and its alloys. Grade 1 commercially pure, Grade 5 Ti-6Al-4Va alloy and Grade 23 Ti-6Al-4Va-ELI alloy are of primary interest in both commercial and medical applications. Grade 23 is slightly more corrosion resistant in sea water than Grade 5. It is very similar to Grade 5 containing exactly the same quantities of principal alloying elements but lower quantities of the trace elements, particularly oxygen. The mechanical properties are given in Table 1.1 below.

Table 1.1 Mechanical properties of Titanium and Some of its Alloys.

Material	Density g/cm^3	Min. Yield Strength MPa 0.2% Offset	Min. Ultimate Strength MPa	Young's Modulus GPa	Endurance Limit MPa	Toughness MPam$^{1/2}$	Hardness RC	Elongation %
Grade 1 Commercially Pure Annealed ASTM F67	4.51	170	240	103	120	70	-	25
Grade 2 Commercially Pure Hot Rolled ASTM F67	4.51	250	460	103	240	75	-	20
Grade 23 Ti-6Al-4Va-ELI ASTM F136 Annealed	4.42	450	625	114	320	70	30	25
Grade 23 Ti-6Al-4Va-ELI ASTM F136 H900	4.42	760	828	114	450	75-90	36	10-20

On the basis of weight, heat treated titanium alloys are stronger than any other metal. They can be as strong as hardened steel but weigh 45% less. They are stronger than cobalt alloys and also weigh much less. They are much more flexible than either stainless steels or cobalt alloys thus providing greater mechanical compatibility with bone.

Wrought Titanium alloys are precipitation hardenable. Precipitation hardenable metal is heat treated and quenched prior to release of the material for sale. This produces an alloy with a hardness of about RC35 which can be readily machined with current cutting tools. In these multi phase metals quenching stops phase transformation so that the equilibrium phases do not completely form. After machining the part is then heated at a temperature far below the original heat treatment for, typically, several hours. This heat treatment is called aging. During aging very fine crystals of the trapped phase will precipitate out. These fine crystals inhibit slippage in the much larger crystals from which precipitation occurred thereby increasing the strength and hardness of the metal.

Titanium alloys are reasonably hard but substantially inferior in hardness and abrasion resistance to hardened steels or Vitallium. They are thus, subject to fretting corrosion where there is micro motion between contacting parts and wear of the counterface of an articulating metal against plastic articulating couple. Fortunately, this weakness can be overcome by coating the titanium substrates with a thin film ceramic, such as titanium nitride (TiN), which is much harder than cobalt alloys [6-8].

Finally, Titanium and its alloys are not ferromagnetic. Thus, they do not interfere with CT scans as do the Co-Cr alloys which are ferromagnetic.

c) Biocompatibility

Titanium is a very reactive metal. Fortunately, it quickly reacts with oxygen to form, self healing, hard titanium oxide film which inhibits corrosion. Thus, titanium is the most corrosion resistant non noble metal approaching the overall corrosion resistance of platinum. It is particularly corrosion resistant to sea water as is its Ti-6Al-4Va-ELI alloy used in medical applications [5]. This superior corrosion resistance produces a high level of biocompatibility.

Further, titanium ions are not toxic even in large quantities [2]. It is estimated that almost a milligram of titanium is ingested by humans each day but most is excreted without being absorbed.

The authors have noted in the retrieval of titanium and Co-Cr Implants fixed by biological ingrowth that titanium ingrowth occurs over almost the entire fixation surfaces and that there is direct contact between the titanium and bone. Ingrowth on the Co-Cr alloy fixation surfaces, on the other hand, is limited to a few small areas, like "spot welding". Even in these areas microscopic examination shows no direct contact of Co-Cr alloy and bone, but rather, a thin fibrous tissue layer is interposed between metal and bone. Titanium and its alloys are the most biocompatible of the materials used for orthopaedic implants.

1.5.1.2 Cobalt Chromium Alloys

a) Introduction

Cobalt alloys have been used in the body at least since the 1930's, after an alloy called Vitallium, a variation of the alloy called "Haynes Stellite" was developed in the 1920's. There are three types of cobalt alloys in general use. There are wear resistant, temperature resistant and corrosion resistant alloys. This section will deal only with the corrosion resistant alloys, such as Vitallium.

Parts made from such alloys were generally made as investment castings since originally it was not practical to machine such alloys due to their hardness and brittleness. Recently, however, wrought alloys, cutting tools and methods have been developed so that now machining of cobalt alloys is practical. Parts are routinely now machined from cobalt alloys. Still the cost of Co-Cr parts is relatively high when one considers the combined effects of the costs of materials processing.

b) Physical Properties

Cobalt, like titanium has a hexagonal crystal structure at room temperature. At elevated temperatures the crystal structure becomes face centered cubic. Thus, the addition of alloying elements can produce a multi phase material and make possible precipitation hardening allowing, with proper processing, high strength and hardness [9]. The stiffness and density of these alloys are similar to those of stainless steels. Thus they do not offer the advantages of lower stiffness and weight for use in implants associated with titanium. The principal advantage of Co-Cr alloys is their very high hardness and abrasion resistance. Thus these materials make an excellent counterface material in a metal against plastic articulating couple.

As cast material, as originally used in orthopaedics, Co-Cr alloys are substantially inferior in strength to other implant metals. More recently post casting processing, such as the Hot Isostatic Press (HIP) process substantially improves the strength of Co-Cr alloys to the point where they approach that of Titanium [10].

Such improvement is necessary to minimize the risk of implant fractures [11]. Still the risk of intergranular corrosion leading to fracture [12] is significant unless the casting and post casting processes are very well controlled.

c) Biocompatibility

Cobalt alloys have been used successfully for implants for more than a half century. Clearly, then, they have an acceptable level of biocompatibility. This biocompatibility, as in the case of titanium, stems from the formation of a hard oxide film. Since cobalt is not as reactive as titanium this film is not as quick in formation and is not as self healing. It does not provide corrosion protection equal to the oxide film on titanium. As a result some small degree of corrosion, and therefore, metal ion release takes place from Co-Cr implants.

These corrosion products are, to some degree, toxic and can provoke an allergic reaction [13-16]. It has been observed by the authors that bone will not always grow against Co-Cr alloys. There is usually a fibrous tissue layer between Co-Cr and bone in vivo.

1.5.1.3 Stainless Steel

a) Introduction
Steel is an iron – carbon alloy. A simplified iron – carbon equilibrium diagram is shown in Fig. 1.6 [1].

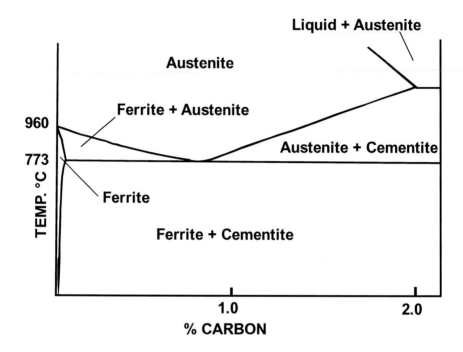

Fig. 1.6 A Simplified Iron – Carbon Equilibrium Diagram.

At room temperature it is a two phase alloy called "pearlite", consisting mostly of "ferrite", which has a body centered cubic crystal structure and is magnetic, and "cementite" a compound of iron and carbon. At high enough temperatures the material becomes a single phase, "austenite", which is face centered cubic and non magnetic. The amount of cementite increases with the amount of carbon. The corrosion resistance of steel declines with an increase in carbon content since there is more of the second phase to promote corrosion.

Moderate and high (.04-1.0%) carbon steels may be hardened by heating at temperatures in the austenitic region and then very rapid cooling (quenching) to room temperature. This can produce steels with an ultimate strength in excess of 1000 MPa and a hardness of RC65. The resulting microstructure is called "martensite". Such materials are then, usually heated at a temperature midway between melting and room temperature for several hours (tempered) to minimize the internal stresses and the brittle behavior of the "as quenched" material.

Other alloying elements are used to, alter the phase transition regions so as to improve the results of heat treatment, improve mechanical properties and, particularly, corrosion resistance. The focus here will be on the latter. A substantial amount of chromium is used for all stainless steels since these steels develop a passive chromium oxide thin film which provides the bulk of the corrosion protection. Nickel is used to extend the austenite range so that the material is single phase at room temperature also improving corrosion resistance since the presence of multiple phases promotes corrosion due to the difference in electrical potential between phases.

To maximize corrosion resistance of stainless steels it is desirable to passivate (chemically clean) all parts of such material to remove impurities from the surface deposited during processing and handling.

There are more than 60 grades of stainless steels in six series available today. Of interest in orthopaedic use are the 300 series of austenitic chromium-nickel steel, the 400 series of ferrite, martensitic alloys and the 630-635 series of semi austenitic, martensitic precipitation hardening alloys [17].

1) Austenitic (300 series)

These are the original 18-8 (18%Cr-8%Ni) stainless steels. Since they are single phase alloys they cannot be hardened by heat treatment. They can, however be hardened by cold working to achieve very high strength. Of interest in orthopaedics is the 316L alloy, a low carbon variation with molybdenum added to improve corrosion resistance in sea water [18].

Such alloys have been in clinically successful use as implants for many decades. They are much lower in cost than other orthopaedic metals. Still the far superior corrosion properties of titanium alloys and other orthopaedic metals should almost stop the use of stainless steels as implants. Other, stronger, less expensive, stainless steels are better suited for instrument use.

2) Ferritic (400) series

These stainless steels are not sufficiently corrosion resistant for implant use. They are, however, sufficiently corrosion resistant for instrument use where the corrosive environments are long term room storage or short term autoclave conditions. These steels are hardenable and the hardness and strength available in such steels makes them of value for orthopaedic instruments. This is particularly the case where great abrasion resistance, such as in cutting guide surfaces, is important. A good general purpose steel of the type is the 420 grade which is often used in cutlery. A higher carbon 440 alloy may also be useful where additional hardness is needed and some corrosion resistance can be sacrificed.

3) Precipitation Hardening (600 series)

These alloys are used entirely for instruments. A common alloy is 17-4 PH where the 17 and 4 are symbolic of the percent of chromium and nickel and PH is symbolic of precipitation hardening [19]. The ability to harden the material after machining at temperatures far below the temperatures associated with the hardening of carbon steel or the 400 series alloys and the elimination of the need for quenching and tempering makes parts made of these alloys simple and inexpensive to heat treat without the distortion and dimensional changes often associated with the heat treatment of steels [1].

1.5.1.4 Aluminum

Due to its light weight, low cost and reasonable corrosion resistance aluminum may be useful for orthopaedic instruments. In pure form it is quite corrosion resistant but of low strength. Alloys sacrifice corrosion resistance for increased strength due to precipitation hardening. Many alloys of differing strength, cost and corrosion resistance are available. The most commonly used alloy is 6061T6 which has yield strength of about 230MPa and fatigue strength of about 110MPa. This is about ¼ the strength of titanium alloy [1].

Aluminum is useful for instrument parts not requiring high strength or hardness such as handles, spacers, etc. Aluminum parts should be clear anodized to minimize degradation of surface appearance due to corrosion.

1.5.1.5 Zirconium

Zirconium is another highly reactive metal that like titanium is highly corrosion resistant due to the formation of an oxide film [20]. Its elastic modulus is similar to titanium but it is substantially inferior in strength and weighs 50% more [21]. It has low toxicity but can cause skin irritation in powder form [22]. Like titanium, zirconium can be anodized to created a thicker than natural oxide film [23]. This zirconium oxide film is, however, thinner than the ceramic TiN film used with titanium and not as hard.

Although apparently inferior to titanium in implant applications it is also significantly more costly and thus, seems of limited use in orthopaedics. Its principal use is for its superior corrosion resistance to certain industrial chemicals in situations where this corrosion resistance is worth the extra cost.

1.5.2 Polymers

Plastics have been in orthopaedic use for more than half a century. Several plastics, such as Teflon and Delrin, were tried in joint replacement. Finally, Charnley and Craven [24] applied Ultra high molecular weight polyethylene (UHMWPe) to the Charnley hip replacement in 1962 and it became the dominant, if not sole, plastic used in orthopaedic joint replacements.

1.5.2.1 UHMWPe

a) Introduction
UHMWPe is a thermosetting plastic that is a subset of the thermoplastic polyethylene. Thermosetting plastics are so viscous after melting that they cannot be processed by injection molding. Thermoplastic plastics can be injection molded.

It is a high performance plastic that, despite its relatively weak Van der Waals bonds, which produce the strength of most strong plastics such as Kevlar, derives sufficient strength from its extremely long individual molecules. UHMWPe has extremely long polymer chains with a molecular weight usually between 2 and 6 million. It is an extremely tough material with a low coefficient of friction and very high abrasion resistance.

Unfortunately, the weak Van der Waals bonding results in a material which has relatively poor resistance to heat. Fortunately, it has very low water absorption, is highly corrosion resistant and non toxic. As a result it is an excellent material for bearings in orthopaedic joint replacement where its positive factors are important but heat resistance is not.

b) Physical Properties
Reference [25] provides a description and data on the physical properties of UHMWPe. At +23C the tensile yield strength is about 20MPa. There is no data provided on the more important compressive yield. Testing performed during the study of Ref. [26], however indicates that the compressive yield strength is about 30MPa. Young's modulus at +23C is about 700MPa but at body temperature it decreases to about 600MPa. No data on tensile fatigue is provided in [25] but compressive fatigue appears to be about 10MPa.

UHMWPe has a density of about 0.93.

c) Biocompatibility
In bulk form UHMWPe is inert and non toxic in vivo. Although UHMWPe is highly wear resistant it is not wear free. Fine wear particles, with their very large surface area to volume ratio, do, however, as they do in metals, produce adverse biological effects in vivo [27]. These include osteolysis and cyst formation. Such problems are the limiting factor in the longevity of joint replacements.

d) Improved UHMWPe
Over the last two decades efforts have been made to improve the wear performance of UHMWPe. With, perhaps, the exception of additional cross linking, all have failed. The first was the addition of carbon fiber to the polyethylene by Zimmer, a major orthopaedic device manufacturer. This attempt failed, probably due to the poor bonding of the polyethylene to the carbon fibers.

Later, DePuy, another major device manufacturer, in collaboration with DuPont developed and introduced a more highly crystalline form called "Hylamer". Although some attributed its poor performance to the oxidizing effects of gamma radiation [28], knee simulator testing [29] and oscillating pin-on-disk testing [30] comparing Hylamer with conventional UHMWPe showed greatly increased wear in the Hylamer (a four times increase) with unsterilized materials.

Further, the most serious wear problems occur in knee devices. Here the incongruity of most such devices made the increased stiffness of Hylamer a serious disadvantage.

Highly cross linked UHMWPe was clinically introduced in the late 1990's. It has gained wide acceptance, at least in the USA. These materials are cross linked, for orthopaedic applications, by gamma or electron beam irradiation. Such radiation unfortunately, greatly reduces the corrosion resistance of UHMWPe, particularly oxidation resistance. This can substantially degrade the in vivo performance of the material. Further, both oxidation and radiation greatly reduce the ductility of the material substantially increasing the risk of crack formation and fatigue failure.

To overcome these problems most highly cross-linked UHMWPe is annealed in an effort to drive off the free radicals inducing oxidation and to improve ductility. To what degree such heat treatment reduces cross linking and wear resistance is not clear, but likely it will reduce them to some degree. An excellent review of the effects of radiation on UHMWPe is found in Ref. [31].

Recently the incorporation of vitamin E into the UHMWPe before irradiation seems to limit the adverse effects of irradiation, at least with regard to the reduction in oxidation resistance. It does nothing, however, to improve ductility. Chemical cross linking is used primarily in industry to improve the properties of UHMWPe. It avoids many of the problems associated with irradiation. Why it is not used for orthopaedic devices is not discussed. It is likely due to concerns as to the biocompatibility of the materials as chemically modified.

The increase in stiffness and tendency toward crack formation and reduced fatigue resistance resulting from irradiation makes the application of such materials to incongruent knee designs, common in the USA, worrisome. Fortunately, the wear in congruent, mobile bearing knees with their large contact areas and low contact stresses seems low enough that wear improvement in such knees is unnecessary [32].

Although it seems likely that highly cross-linked UHMWPe improves wear properties there are still some question as to the extent of such improvement. Simulator studies performed by, or with the support of, orthopaedic device manufacturers show wear reductions that are modest and in some cases unbelievable. Testing by the authors shows an increase in wear due to radiation in both pin-on-disk and hip simulator. In a simulator study, using the hip simulator illustrated in Fig. 1.7, using randomly variable figure 8 wear tracks, acetabular bearings radiated at 2.5MRa, the normal sterilization dose, showed about a 50% increase in wear compared to conventional UHMWPe.

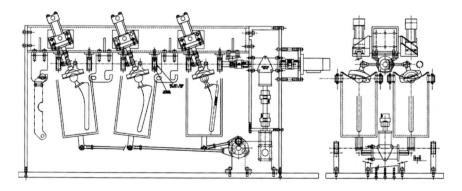

Fig. 1.7 B-P Six Station Hip Simulator.

It has been the experience of the authors that there seems little correlation between simulator wear and wear in vivo. For example, in a 48M hip simulation [33] TiN coated femoral heads showed negligible wear that was only a small fraction of the wear by Co-Cr heads. In clinical use, however, the penetration observed with TiN coated heads was not significantly different than those observed with Co-Cr heads.

In the case of highly cross-linked UHMWPe one does see a significant, but modest, reduction in penetration [28]. This reduction may, however, not entirely be due to a reduction in wear. Under stress UHMWPe is subject to permanent deformation due to loading called "creep". Radiation significantly increases the hardness and stiffness, and thus, likely the creep resistance of UHMWPe. Thus most, if not all of the reduction in penetration may be due to creep and not wear reduction.

Meanwhile there are reports of problems with cross linked UHMWPe [34] since most manufacturers claim proprietary and different processes; probably with different performance properties it will be difficult to access the overall performance of cross - linked polyethylene.

1.5.2.2 Acetals

Acetal is the usual name for a family of PolyOxyMethylene thermoplastics. There are two basic forms: copolymer and monopolymer. The most commonly known and used variation is "Delrin" a monopolymer developed by DuPont in the early 1950's. Copolymers are widely available from a variety of sources.

As a plastics group Acetals have high stiffness, strength, dimensional stability with good wear and frictional properties, good corrosion resistance and low water absorption. Monopolymers generally have somewhat greater mechanical properties but slightly lesser corrosion resistance than copolymers [35].

Delrin was used clinically in the 1960's as a joint replacement bearing material [36] because of its excellent strength, wear and frictional properties. It was abandoned, however, notwithstanding the favorable biocompatibility testing of Ref. 35, since DuPont felt it could leach formaldehyde and thus, they would not sell it for use in humans.

Still Acetals are of value in surgical instruments, particularly trials since they have sufficient heat and corrosion resistance with low water absorption and thus, can withstand repeated autoclaving. They are commonly used on impact surfaces to avoid damage to the impacted part and as joint replacement bearing trials. They are generally cheaper and easier to machine than most metals used in instruments.

1.5.2.3 Others

Many other engineering plastics are available and are of potential use in orthopaedics. Several have been used in instruments and trials but they are generally of higher cost and generally inferior in overall mechanical and chemical properties to the Acetals.

1.5.3 Surface Modification

Coatings and other surface modification means such as nitriding, carbonizing, anodizing and passivation have been used in industry to improve the corrosion and wear properties of metals for more than a century. Most have also been used to some degree for orthopaedic implants and instruments.

1.5.3.1 Passivation

Passivation is essentially a cleaning process to remove any scale or impurities from the surfaces of a part usually by some acid.   Such processes can substantially improve surface corrosion resistance by eliminating surface contaminants introduced during the manufacture of the part. These contaminates may themselves corrode and produce local galvanic cells accelerating surface corrosion. It is essential that all orthopaedic devices be passivated prior to distribution.

1.5.3.2 Porous Coating

Biological fixation is, or should be, the normal means of attaching metallic implants to bone. It avoids the problems associated with cement [37, 38] and is less expensive to use. There are many ways to obtain a porous fixation surface. Among these are:

(a) Sintered Bead
Here gas-atomized spherical beads are sintered on to the metal part substrate. Differing size beads produce differing pore sizes with a porosity of about 35%. Commercially pure titanium beads are used for titanium alloy implants and Co-Cr beads for Co-Cr implants. Such a coating is shown in Fig. 1.8.

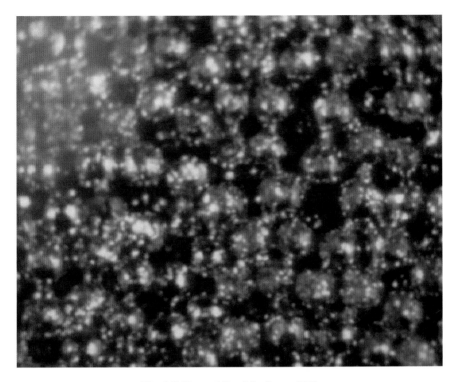

Fig. 1.8 Sintered Bead Surface – 50X.

These coatings have been in successful use for more than thirty years and are still widely used today. Unfortunately, the high temperature sintering process adversely affects the mechanical properties of the metal to which it is applied. Sintering temperatures approach the melting point of the substrate. Local melting of the points of contact between beads, however, occurs before the substrate material melts. This high temperature substantially reduces (by about one third) the strength of the substrate by increasing grain growth. Further, the addition of the beads creates local stress magnification due to the stress concentration effect of the small radii at the bead connections. Thus, the strength of the part is generally reduced to about only one-third of its original strength by the addition of a sintered bead porous coating. Further, sintered bead parts cannot be precipitation hardened.

Still by not coating areas of critical stress thus keeping stress below these lower values of failure stress the loss in strength can be accommodated by proper design. An example may be seen in Fig. 1. 9.

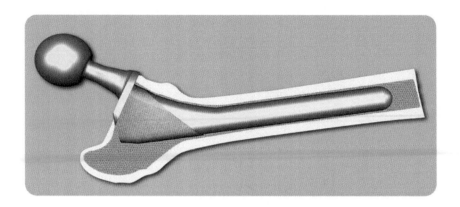

Fig. 1.9 B-P Femoral Stem with Partial Porous Coating.

It may be seen that at midstem where stresses are highest there is an absence of porous coating. Here the stem has still lost 1/3 of its strength but not the full 2/3 loss associated with this coating. Such a situation is not true for a ¾ length coated stem, or even most proximally coated stems where the entire strength loss is encountered. Fortunately, the metals used for most stems can be capable of supporting the expected loading.

The control of the process used to apply such coatings must be very robust and precise. Careful inspection of the coated parts is essential. The authors have observed several instances of defective coatings including the delamination of such coatings and the shedding of its beads leading to failure of the joint replacement.

(b) Other Porous Coatings

Several other methods of producing a porous metal surface have been developed and used. These include: Plasma spray, fiber mesh, porous metal [39] and, more recently chemical surface etching [40] and electro-discharge machining (EDM)].

In the plasma process titanium is sprayed onto a substrate, not necessarily titanium, in a reduced pressure inert gas chamber at high temperature producing an irregularly shaped porous surface. Flame parameters and the composition of the powder determine the nature of the irregularities. Bonding of the coating to the substrate is generally inferior than developed by sintered bead coating since adhesion, rather than ionic bonding occurs in plasma sprayed coatings.

Fiber mesh and porous titanium are similar to sintered bead coating except in the case of fiber mesh fibers and in the case of porous titanium a titanium sponge is used rather than beads. The adverse effects of such coatings on titanium are similar to sintered bead coatings. Where such coating is used on Co-Cr alloy parts one also has the effect of lower bond strength as in the case of plasma spray coatings. These latter methods produce a greater porosity than sintered bead ranging from 50-70% [39].

The most promising are the recent development of porous coating produced by selective chemical etching of the substrate and the deposition of a porous coating by EDM. With these methods there are no adverse thermal effects. Parts strengthen by heat treatment are not affected other than by the stress concentration effects of the pores. Such parts can be at least twice as strong as sintered bead coated parts.

1.5.3.3 Hydroxyapatite

Hydroxyapatite (HA) is a bioactive ceramic coating used on both titanium and Co-Cr alloy implants to promote bone ingrowth onto the implants. It is clear that HA produces more rapid ingrowth and increases bond strength to bone with Co-Cr implants. There is, however, no significant strength increase in the long-term when it is used on titanium [41].

As in most materials and coatings the single advantage of HA is offset by several disadvantages. HA is a hard, brittle calcium phosphate ceramic with intrinsically poor mechanical properties [42]. It relies on the support of the substrate material for support. Even when applied to a porous implant the 3D interlocking of HA and metal only improves on the poor adhesive bond strength and not on the poor shear resistance of HA. Further, little is known about the fatigue of HA, but one would expect poor fatigue resistance particularly since the material is attacked and resorbed by the body. Static bond strength tests indicate little about the fatigue properties of HA and, thus, its long term mechanical performance in the body.

Such coatings are usually applied by plasma flame spray at very high temperatures degrading the mechanical properties of the substrate. In addition fatigue inducing tensile stresses are created on the metallic part by the differences in the coefficients of thermal expansion further degrading the part to which the HA coating is applied. Newer coating processes and coating materials are under development in a effort to reduce these adverse effects [43, 44] and one would expect to see better HA coatings in the future.

The main problem is that HA coatings provide only marginal advantages over uncoated implants and increase the cost of such implants. This is particularly true for titanium implants where bone apposition is relatively rapid and complete over the porous implant surfaces. In the current, tightly, cost - controlled market, an increase in cost for an improvement that cannot be demonstrated clinically, even ignoring potential problems associated with the disadvantages noted, may not be justified.

1.5.3.4 Ceramic Films

In addition to improvements in the plastic element of an articulating couple in orthopaedic joint replacement, improvements in the counterface element are also of value. The use of ceramic films is one means of obtaining such improvement. There are many ceramic films that are potential candidates for such improvement. Among these are CrN for use on Co-Cr implants, diamond like, and titanium nitride (TiN) and it's much harder variations titanium aluminum nitride (TiAlN) and titanium carbon nitride (TiCN) [45] which are best used on titanium. Zirconium Oxide (ZrO) is used on zirconium implants.

(a) Titanium Nitride
TiN is, by far, the most widely used implant coating material. It is an extremely hard ceramic which is also strong and biologically inert. It is used to improve the wear resistance of cutting tools and sliding surfaces. It has been used on dental implants for several decades and on orthopaedic implants for the last two decades.

TiN is usually applied to titanium alloys by a physical vapor deposition (PVD) process by sputter deposition, cathodic arc deposition or electron beam heating. In cathodic arc deposition the parts to be coated are placed in a vacuum chamber with pure titanium cathodes as illustrated in Fig. 1.10.

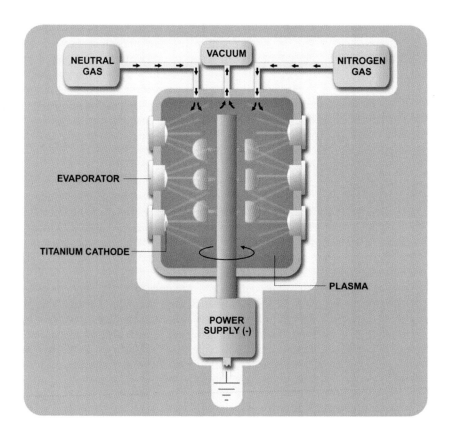

Fig. 1.10 TiN Applied by PVD Cathodic Arc Deposition.

A high vacuum is drawn, a neutral gas is fed into the chamber and an electrical plasma arc struck. Titanium ions are expelled at high speed from the cathode and deposited on the parts to be coated. Nitrogen gas is then slowly fed into the chamber. Some of the titanium ions then combine with the nitrogen to produce TiN which is then also deposited resulting in a very thin transition layer of combined titanium and titanium nitride. Ultimately, all the titanium ions expelled from the cathode are converted to TiN resulting in the final TiN coating as illustrated in Fig. 1.11.

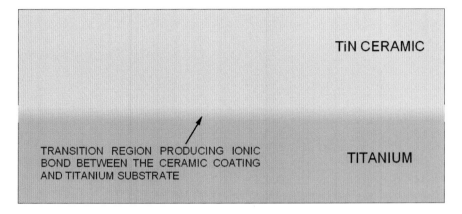

Fig. 1.11 Cross Section of Tin Coating.

Since the substrate is titanium and the transition layer gradually changes from pure titanium to TiN the bond between layers is ionic rather than adhesive as it is for other substrates or coatings. Ionic bonding is such that the surface bond is much stronger than is the case of an adhesive bond.

Although a TiN counterface does not have a substantially lower coefficient of friction than Co-Cr alloy, since it is much harder it is not as readily degraded by the effects of articulation. Thus, it does not increase significantly with time as illustrated in Fig. 1.12.

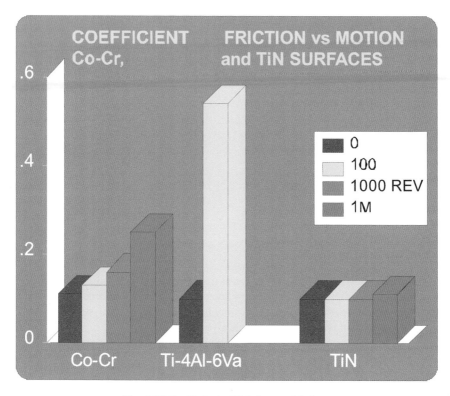

Fig. 1.12 Coefficient of Friction vs. Motion

The apparatus used to conduct the experiment of Fig 1.12 is shown in Fig. 1.13.

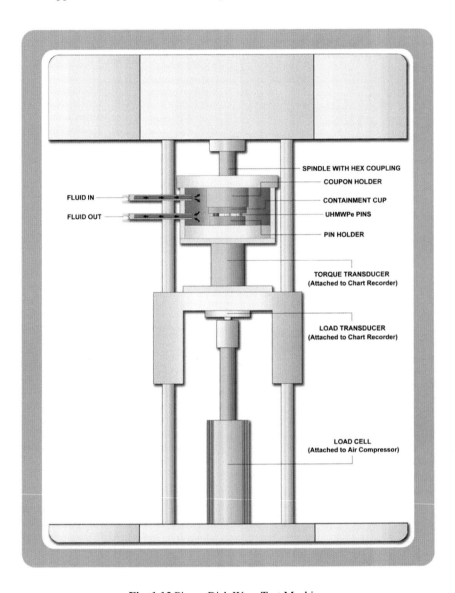

Fig. 1.13 Pin on Disk Wear Test Machine.

The author's work [33] found lower wear for TiN than Co-Cr in a hip simulator test of laboratory prepared femoral heads as may be seen in Fig. 1.14.

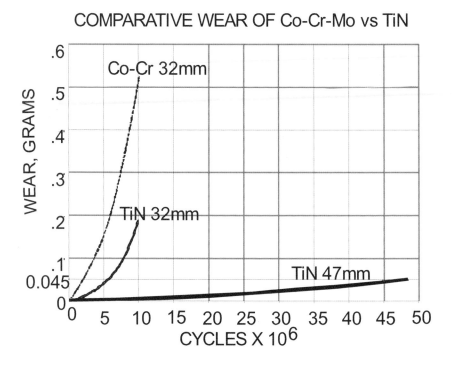

Fig. 1.14 Wear in a Hip Simulator Comparing TiN and Co-Cr vs. UHMWPe.

Unfortunately, the promise of much lower wear was not borne out in clinical experience or in the test of production prostheses where wear was approximately similar for both TiN coated and Co-Cr devices [46, 47]. The difference in performance between the laboratory prepared and production samples is likely due to differences in surface finish. The studies of both [45] and [46] found that for the production parts tested the parts coated with TiN were substantially rougher then the Co-Cr alloy parts. Test by the authors found that production TiN coated parts had a surface roughness of about 15μin Ra. The laboratory samples used in the simulator test had a surface finish of about 0.5 μin Ra. This difference can produce an order of magnitude wear change as illustrated by Dowson [48] in Fig. 1.15.

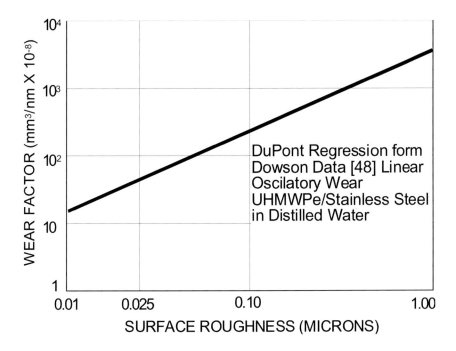

Fig. 1.15 Wear vs. Surface Roughness [48].

The superior properties of titanium for orthopaedic implants can be fully exploited by the use of ceramic TiN coating by converting a material with relatively poor abrasion and wear resistance to a material with superior abrasion and wear resistance. Endotec, a small orthopaedic implant device manufacturer, has applied the benefits to all its joint replacement products, illustrated in Fig. 1.16, for the last two decades

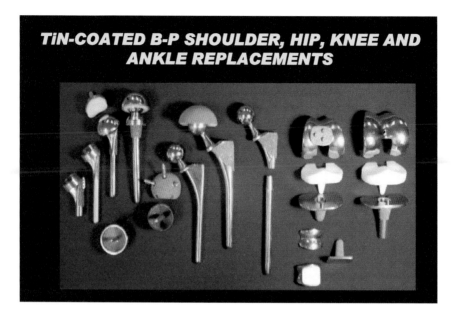

Fig. 1.16 Endotec Line of Titanium Alloy Ceramic Coated Implants.

(b) Oxides

As mentioned in the sections on titanium and zirconium these materials can be anodized, i.e. artificially oxidized by heating and immersion in an oxidizing environment, to produce a 5 micron thick oxide coating thereby increasing abrasion and wear resistance and reducing UHMWPe wear in an articulating couple. Such oxide layers are, however, inferior in mechanical properties to nitrides and thus find limited use in orthopaedics. Further, such oxidation tends to destroy porous surfaces and, as a consequence, anodized devices do not allow biological fixation further limiting their use.

(c) Others

Both titanium and Co-Cr alloys can be surfaces hardened by "Nitriding", that is adding nitrogen ions onto their surface by several means as has been done for hardening steels for the last century. The resulting surface is improved but is inferior to Nitride films such as TiN.

1.6 Conclusion

Orthopaedic materials are primarily decades old, developed for general application. Early attempts to develop materials specifically for orthopaedic use have generally failed. Even the current development of highly cross linked UHMWPe is an extension of the development of such materials outside of the orthopaedic establishment for general use.

References

[1] Diagram, E.P.: Materials and Processes in Manufacturing, Ch. 2. MacMillan Publishing Co., New York (1974)

[2] Black, J.: Biological Performance of Materials - Fundamentals of Biocompatibility. Marcel Dekker, New York (1981)

[3] Corrosion: Wikipedia CD Selection (2006), http://schools-wikipedia.org/2006/wp/c/Corrosion.htm (accessed August 27,2009)

[4] Fernandez-Fairen, M., et al.: Aging of Retrieved Zirconia Femoral Heads. Clinical Orthopaedics and Related Research 462, 122–129 (2007)

[5] Titanium, http://en.wikipedia.org/wiki/Titanium (accessed August 29, 2009)

[6] Titanium nitride, http://en.wikipedia.org/wiki/Titanium_nitride (accessed August 29, 2009)

[7] Bolster, R.N., et al.: Tribological Behavior of TiN Films Deposited by High Energy. Ion-Beam-Assisted Deposition, Surface and Coatings Technology 36, 105–116 (1988)

[8] Johansen, O.A., et al.: Reactive Arc Vapor Ion Deposition of TiN, ZrN, and HfN. Thin Solid Films 153 (1987)

[9] Cast Nonferrous: Cobalt and Cobalt Alloys, http://keytometals.com/Article54.htm (accessed August 26, 2009)

[10] Harris, K., Sicken, S.: Investment Cast Cobalt Alloys (2007), http://www.c-mgroup.com/abstracts/investment_cast_alloys.htm (accessed August 28, 2009))

[11] Woolson, S.T., et al.: Fatigue Fracture of Forged Cobalt-Chromium-Molybdenum Femoral Component Inserted with Cement - A Report of ten Cases. Journal of Bone and Joint Surgery[Am] 79A(12), 1842–1848 (1997)

[12] Gilbert, J.L., et al.: Intergranular Corrosion-Fatigue Failure of Cobalt-Alloy Femoral Stems. A Failure Analysis of Two Cases. Journal of Bone and Joint Surgery [Am] 76A(1), 110–115 (1994)

[13] Black, J.: Biological Performance of Materials - Fundamentals of Biocompatibility, ch.12. Marcel Dekker, New York (1981)

[14] Gawkrodger, D.J.: Metal Sensitivities and Orthopaedic Implants Revisited: The Potential Metal Allergy with New Metal-on-Metal Prostheses. British Journal of Dermatology 148(6), 1089–1093 (2005) ISSN: 0007-0963

[15] Saglam, A.M., et al.: Nickel and Cobalt hypersensitivity Reaction Before and After Orthodontic Therapy in Children. Journal of Contemporary Dental Practice 5(4), 1526–3711 (2004)

[16] Goon, A.T., Goh, C.L.: Metal Allergy in Singapore. Contact Dermatitis 52(3), 130–132, 105–1873 (2004) ISSN: 0105-1873

[17] Properties of Stainless Steel Alloys, http://www.aerdynealloys.com/stainless-steel-alloy-properties.php (accessed August 28, 2009)

[18] High Grade Machinable Type 316L Steel, http://www.smithmetal.com (accessed August 27, 2009)

[19] Precipitation Hardening Stainless Steel bar, http://www.smithmetal.com (accessed August 27, 2009)

[20] Zirconium (Zr) Material Information,
      http://gooffellow.com/A/Zirconium.html
      (accessed September 2, 2009)

[21] News 19.8.09: titanium Alloy Ti-13Nb-12Zr Round Bar ASTM F1713 > > zirconium
      702/705 ASME Allowable Stress, http://titanex.com/zr/zirkonium-
      zircone.php?sel+3 (accessed September 2, 2009)

[22] Zirconium, http://www.ithyroid.com/sirconium.htm
      (accessed September 2, 2009)

[23] Zirconium Alloy Data Sheet. bulletin A/12c, Flowserve Corp., Dayton Ohio (June
      1989)

[24] Ultra High Molecular Weight Polyethylene,
      http://en.wilipedia.org/wikw/Ultra_high_molecular_weight-
      ployethylene (accessed August 28, 2009)

[25] Hostalen, G.U.R.: Hoechst Aktiengesellschaft, Verkauf Kunstoffe. 6230 Frankfurt
      am Main 80 (1982)

[26] Pappas, M.J., Makris, G., Buechel, F.F.: Contact stresses in metal plastic total knee
      replacements: A theoretical and experimental study. Biomedical Engineering
      Technical Report. Jensen Beach Florida (1986)

[27] Wang, M.L., et al.: Particle Bioreactivity and Wear-Mediated Osteolysis. The Journal
      of Arthroplasty 19(8), 1028–1038 (2004)

[28] Martell, J.M., et al.: Clinical Performance of a Highly Cross-Linked Polyethylene at
      Two Years in Total Hip Arthroplasty: A Randomized Prospective Trial. The Journal
      of Arthroplasty 18(7), 55–59 (2003)

[29] Canonaco, A.: An evaluation of wear characteristics of Hylamer and UHMWPe
      bearings in knee replacement systems under stimulation (Master Thesis). NJIT
      Newark, NJ (1994)

[30] D'Alessio, J.: Wear and friction of Hylamer and UHMWPe against cobalt chromium
      for the evaluation of use in the manufacturing of orthopaedic implants (Master
      Thesis). NJIT Newark, NJ (1994)

[31] Shaw, J.H.: The Effect of Gamma Irradiation on Ultra High Molecular Weight
      Polyethylene - A Review of the Literature to November 1996. Medical Devices
      Agency, UK Department of Health, London (1997)

[32] Buechel Sr., F.F., Buechel Jr., F.F., Helbig, T.E., Pappas, M.J.: "31 year evolution of
      the rotating-platform TKR: Coping with "spin-out" and wear". Presented at the
      ASTM Symposium on Mobile Bearing Total Knee Replacement Devices, St Louis,
      May 18 (2010)

[33] Pappas, M.J., Makris, G., Buechel, F.F.: Titanium Nitride Ceramic Film Against
      Polyethylene: a 48 Million Cycle Test. Clinical Orthopaedics and Related
      Research 317, 64–70 (1995)

[34] Bradford, L., et al.: Wear and Surface Cracking in early Retrieved Highly Cross-
      Linked Polyethylene Acetabular Liners. Journal of Bone and Joint Surgery[Am] 86A,
      1271–1281 (2004)

[35] Acetal (Poly-Oxy-Methylene) Specifications,
      http://www.boedeker.com.acetalp.htm (accessed August 28, 2009)

[36] Dumbleton, J.H.: Delrin as a Material for Joint Prostheses - A Review. Corrosion and
      Degradation of Implant Materials. In: Syrett, B.C., Acharya, A. (eds.) ASTM STP,
      vol. 684, pp. 41–60. ASTM (1979)

[37] Willert, H.G., Semlitsh, M.: Reaction of the articular capsule to wear products of artificial joint prostheses. Journal of Biomedical Materials Research 11, 134–164 (1977)

[38] Gelante, J.O., et al.: The Biological Effects of Implant Materials. Journal Of Orthopaedic Research 9, 760–775 (1991)

[39] CSTI vs Other Porous Coating,
http://www.pacewithlife.com/ctl?template-PC&op+global&action+1&id+9045&template (accessed August 28, 2009)

[40] Wagner II, D.J.: Chemical Texturing. BONEZone, 45–48 (1989) (Spring 2003)

[41] Hayashi, K., et al.: Evaluation of Metal Implants Coated with Several Types of Ceramics as Biomaterials. Journal of The Society for Biomaterials 23, 11 (1989)

[42] Sahay, V.: Characterization of Composite Hydroxyapatite Coatings for Medical and Dental Devices (2007),
http://www.astm.org/DIGITAL_LIBRARY/STP/PAGES/STP25185S.htm (accessed September 4, 2009)

[43] Yamamoto, H., et al.: 3498 bone-Like Thin HA Coating on Titanium Acquires High Osteoconductivity (2009),
http://iadr.confex.com/iadr/2004Hawaii/tech/techprogram/abstract_44536.htm

[44] Nano Hydroxyapatite Coating for Next Generation Prostheses,
http://www.infrmat.com/hydro2.ht (accessed September 4, 2009)

[45] TiCN (Titanium Carbo-Nitride),
http://tincoat.net/coatings/ticn.html
(accessed September 4, 2009)

[46] Jones, V.C., et al.: New Materials for Mobile Bearing Knee Prosthesis - Titanium Nitride Counterface Coatings for Reduction of Polyethylene Wear. In: LCS: Mobile Bearing Knee Arthroplasty - 25 Years of Worldwide Experience, ch. 21. Springer, Heidelberg (2002)

[47] Bell, C.J., Fisher, J.: Simulation of Polyethylene Wear in Ankle Joint Prostheses. Journal if Biomaterials Research Part B: Applied Biomaterials 81B,162, 167 (2007)

[48] Dowson, D., et al.: Influence of counterface topography on the wear ofUHMWPE under wet and dry condifions. In: Lee, H.L (ed.) The Proceedings of the American Chemical Society, Polymer Wear and tis Control. ACS Symp. Ser., vol. 287, pp. 171–187 (1985)

Chapter 2
Failure Modes

Abstract. This chapter discusses the failure of orthopaedic devices, the causes of such failure and methods of predicting various modes of failure. The primary modes of failure are mechanical, chemical and the adverse biological response to implants. Orthopaedic devices may fracture or deform under loads applied in their use. A prediction of the ability of a device to withstand expected loading in the hostile envioronment in which they are used may be predicted from a knowledge of the mechanical and corrosive properties of the materials used and a knowledge of the loading to which they are subjected. Knowing these, stress analysis may be applied, usually the "Finite Element" method, to determine the stresses and strains throughout the body of the device being evaluated. These stresses and strains are then compared to "safe" values by varous criteria. Wear is the primary mechanical failure mode either by wear through of the part or by the adverse biological response to the products of wear. The various forms of wear are discuseed with the means for minimizing such wear. The dominant mode of wear type failure in incongruent knee repacement bearings is actually fatigue of the articular surface due to excessive contact stresses. Stress analysis of typical incongruent (fixed) and congruent (mobile) knee replacment bearings indicates that the fixed bearing knee bearings analysed are grossly overstressed. Only the mobile bearing device that was analysed has acceptable contact stress values. Mechanical testing confirmed this analysis showing much higher wear for the fixed bearing devices with wear increasing with increasing stress.

2.1 Introduction

The safety and reliability of orthopaedic implant systems is of obvious critical importance. Thus, it is essential to understand the modes and processes of failure and degradation of the elements of such systems and to determine the cause of failure when it occurs. Further, in the design of such systems it is essential to predict the risk of failure and degradation in evaluating designs during the design process, correcting design failures after they occur, but certainly before the release of such devices for general use.

A thorough understanding of mechanical failure involves an understanding of the field of stress analysis [1], corrosion and wear [2]. A thorough understanding of stress analysis involves an understanding of material properties and the "Theory of Elasticity" [3]. Modern techniques for predicting the behavior of materials under loading allow reasonable prediction of such behavior if used in light of knowledge of material properties and elasticity theory. Without such knowledge, however, the results can be very misleading. Thus, this chapter will include a discussion of some classical methods which may be used to augment the computer intensive modern, numerical methods.

An understanding of the risks of biological failure is also essential. Such failure may occur in the absence of any damage to the implants by the release of toxic material from an implant by leaching or corrosion [4]. Biological failure, however, is often associated with mechanical problems such as loosening due to bone necrosis resulting from wear, or mechanical subluxation due to component subsidence.

The science associated with failure prediction is very complex and not completely understood. This chapter, therefore, presents a rather simplified view of the concepts of failure analysis. A more complete understanding may be obtained from the references cited.

2.2 Stress Analysis

Stress analysis involves the prediction of stress and strain in a body under loading or thermal effects. Only the effects of loading will be discussed here.

2.2.1 Stress

The stresses discussed in Chapter 1 are referred to as "simple", one dimensional stresses. If one defines a finite plane in or on a body then if the force is perpendicular to the plane the stress resulting from this force is called a "normal" stress. If the force pulls on the body it is a "tensile" stress and if it pushes on a body it is a "compressive" stress. If the force is parallel to the plane then it is called a "shear" stress. The "average stress" is the force divided by area of the plane.

Average stress is, however, of very limited use. More usual is the situation in which the stress varies from point to point within the body. Thus, often, at critical points in the body one needs to estimate the stress on an infinitesimal element of the body. Thus, we will define "stress" as

$$\sigma = \Delta P \div \Delta A \tag{1}$$

Where:

$limit\ \Delta A \rightarrow 0$

ΔA is the area loaded
ΔP is the force on this area
and σ is the stress.

Most important is the prediction of "maximum" stress which is the largest of the stresses in the body under analysis since failure is most likely to initiate at a point where the stress is maximum.

2.2.1.1 Combined 3D Stress

Furthermore, there may be several forces in several different directions acting on a body which is, of course, three dimensional. As a result one is concerned with an estimate of "combined" stresses in the body.

Consider an elemental cube as shown in Fig. 2.1 where the faces of the cube are in the primary planes of an x, y, z coordinate system.

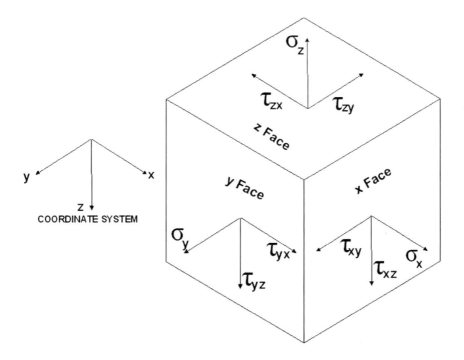

Fig. 2.1 Elemental Cube Showing Stresses on its Faces.

The stress σ_x is the normal stress on x face, τ_{xy} is the shear stress on that face in the y direction etc. In the application of failure theory one is concerned with the "principal" stress in a coordinate system where the shear stresses are zero. These stresses may be found as the roots σ_1, σ_2 and σ_3 of the determinate of the stress matrix:

$$
\begin{vmatrix}
\sigma_x - \sigma & \tau_{xy} & \tau_{xz} \\
\tau_{xy} & \sigma_y - \sigma & \tau_{yz} \\
\tau_{xz} & \tau_{yz} & \sigma_z - \sigma
\end{vmatrix} = 0 \qquad (2)
$$

2.2.1.2 Distortion Energy Theory

Once the principle stresses are known they can be used to predict if these stresses may result in failure, due to these stresses, of the body. Several failure theories have been formulated including the Maximum Normal Stress, Maximum Shear, Strain Energy and the Distortion Energy theories. Each has its strength and weaknesses. Of these theories the most appropriate seems to be the Distortion Energy Theory. This theory compares a combined stress with a safe stress to determine if the combined stress is acceptable. The equation of the comparison is:

$$
\sigma_{eq}^2 = \sigma_1^2 + \sigma_1^2 + \sigma_1^2 - \sigma_1\sigma_2 - \sigma_1\sigma_3 - \sigma_2\sigma_3 \qquad (3)
$$

where σ_{eq} is the equivalent stress, often called the "Von Mises" stress.

2.2.1.3 Soderberg Failure Criterion – Fatigue Failure

Most fractures are the result of a fluctuating load, well below the static failure stresses. Such fluctuating stresses result in "Fatigue" failure. As discussed in Chapter 1 a measure of materials ability to withstand repeated fluctuating stress is its "fatigue strength". Such values usually are determined by a carefully prepared, polished, circular beam sample in a rotating test which subjects the outside surface of the beam to equal compressive and tensile stresses, the most damaging combination. The stress value at which a sample fractures after a given number of cycles, usually 10 million, is the called fatigue strength S_n.

Many parts are not as carefully prepared as a typical fatigue test specimen and allowance must be made for such situations. Thus, the actual fatigue is reduced by factors to account for factors which tend to reduce fatigue strength S_n to a lower value S_m as discussed in Chapter 1.

Further, orthopaedic implants or instruments are not normally subject to complete stress reversal as in the test determining fatigue strength. Thus a safe stress may, in fact, be substantially higher than S_m. A better estimate of an allowable stress may be obtained using the Soderberg Criterion. For example, if the fluctuation is zero for a carefully prepared and polished specimen part failure is assumed to occur at yielding or S_{yp}. If the stress is fluctuating and fully reversed failure is assumed to occur at S_n. Where the fluctuating element is not zero but not fully reversing, the Soderberg Criterion [5] proposes a linear relationship between the extremes as a failure criterion. Thus,

$$
\sigma_f = \sigma_m + \sigma_r S_y/S_n \qquad (4)
$$

Where the mean stress σ_m and the range stress σ_r are:

$$\sigma_m = (\sigma_{max} + \sigma_{min})/2 \qquad (5)$$

$$\sigma_r = (\sigma_{max} - \sigma_{min})/2 \qquad (6)$$

where σ_f is the failure stress, σ_{max} is the maximum stress at a point during the fluctuation and σ_{min} is the minimum stress.

For typical implant or instrument S_n is replaced by S_m and a part is assumed safe against fatigue, if:

$$S_m/N < \sigma_m + \sigma_r S_y/S_m \qquad (7)$$

where N is the factor of safety.

2.2.1.4 Factor of Safety

The factor of safety, occasionally called the factor of ignorance, is used to account for the fact that all estimates of safety against fracture are approximations and in most cases the expected loads are only estimates. Among the factors used are those that reflect the level of control over the materials and manufacturing process used, the accuracy of the computational methods used, the knowledge of what loading to expect and the degree of safety required. Where human safety is involved a factor of safety of 2 is normally used [5].

2.2.2 Stress Computation

In order to use the equations above one must, of course have an estimate of the stresses within or on a body. These stresses are obtained by "Stress Analysis". Classically, designers used either methods based on the Strength of Materials approach or elasticity methods. Today the Strength of Materials approach has little benefit in the analysis of implants since accurate analysis is critical. It can, however, be of use in the analysis of instruments due to the often simple shapes involved. The software package "MathCAD" can be used for such computation and contains a number of subroutines for computation using strength of material methods.

The advent of computer based solid modeling and inexpensive numerical methods based on the theory of elasticity, however, make Finite Element Analysis (FEA), the most commonly used approach. Since this method is based on the classical linear theory of elasticity [3], occasionally modified to include nonlinear effects, an understanding of this theory is essential in understanding the use and results of FEA methodology and software.

2.2.2.1 Classical Theory of Elasticity

In 1821 Navier formulated the basic equations of the theory and Cauchy developed the theory of stress and strain. These were investigated by Saint Venant who used them to solve simple problems of torsion and bending of prismatic bars [3]. As a result of this work Saint Venant formulated the famous Saint Venant principle which allowed for the solution of some practical problems using the theory. The work of these pioneers and others was followed by work by many others leading to the development of the field of applied mechanics which expanded the application of the theory to practical problems.

Unfortunately, the theory establishes a set of simultaneous partial differential equations, constrained by boundary conditions, which cannot, in general, be solved in closed form for the kind of stress determination needed in engineering and particularly in orthopaedic devices. Work in the field of applied mechanics in the early 20th century, however, developed numerical methods for estimating stresses and strains. These methods, although highly labor intensive, were nevertheless used in aircraft design where more accurate estimates were needed to keep weight to a minimum. Such computations often required thousands of man hours to complete.

2.2.2.2 Finite Element Analysis (FEA)

FEA was first introduced in 1943 by Courant using the Ritz numerical method and variational calculus to develop approximate solutions to a class of vibration problems. In 1956, Turner et al expanded the methodology to include the deflection of complex structures [6]. Work over the last half century has greatly expanded the application of FEA and greatly simplified its use.

Linear FEA stress analysis of mechanical parts is now an integral part of most high end computer aided design (CAD) software packages. Although nonlinear FEA analysis is available it is of little practical use in design since it is much more computer intensive and since, in any event, stress in the nonlinear region of almost all materials is to be avoided if failure is to be avoided.

FEA may be used to analyze a mechanical part by creating a digital 3D solid, computer model of the part and then defining a mesh used to approximate the behavior of the part under the expected loading conditions. Such a mesh is shown in Fig. 2.2.

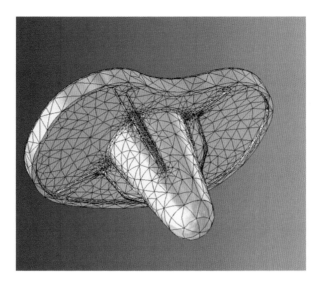

Fig. 2.2 Finite Element Mesh.

Such a mesh consists of a number of points called "nodes". Elements are the material enclosed by the boundary lines connecting the nodes. To perform the analysis an appropriate mesh is first generated with regions of expected high stress and stress concentration using a greater node density. Rigid body constraints are placed on the motion of those nodes where the part is attached to simulate its attachment and forces are placed on appropriate nodes to simulate the expected loading. The resulting problem is then solved computing the approximate stress, and if desired strain, or deformation, at each node. The results are then presented, usually in graphical form to allow easy location of the largest stress and their values.

Although strength of material methods can be used for instruments FEA is a faster and more convenient means of stress and deflection analysis in instruments. This is true since generally 3D solid models are produced during, and as part of, the development of engineering drawings used in the manufacture of such parts. These 3D models are of great importance in the development of surgical and sales brochures and animations or other places where illustrations are used. This same model can also be used in the CAD package in which it was created to perform a relatively accurate FEA estimate of its behavior.

The analysis of implants is another matter. Since the implant is attached to tissue one cannot use rigid body constraints that are normally used without loss of significant accuracy. Further, particularly in the case of femoral stems, one wishes to understand the effect of the applied loads and prosthetic device on the bone onto, or into, which the device has been implanted.

Ideally then, one would create a 3D solid model of the implant attached to a 3D model of the bone in order to perform the analysis. Such an analysis was performed by Crowell [7] who studied an early B-P Ankle Replacement. He found an overstressed region in the tibial plate of the device resulting in a design change increasing its thickness.

Where bone remodeling is of concern one can then proceed with further analysis using a bone remodeling law to alter the properties of the bone model using the stresses found in the bone in the initial analysis. The analysis is then repeated with the remodeled bone. The process is further repeated until the results converge. Such a study was performed by Yau [8] who studied the interaction between Co-Cr and Titanium alloy femoral stems and the proximal femur into which they were implanted.

Unfortunately few designers have sufficient skills, or access to such skills, to fully exploit FEA in implant design. As a result most design decisions are made by comparisons to successful devices or by mechanical tests which often provide a poor, although usually conservative, simulation.

2.3 Mechanical Testing

The approximations used in analysis during design verification often make mechanical and clinical testing a requirement of validation studies. Mechanical test methodology is well defined by a number of American Society for Testing Materials (ASTM) testing protocols developed by industry and the society. Thus, it is usual to use these methods during the mechanical testing phases of verification and validation. Often mechanical testing using these methods is required by regulatory authorities before approval of a device for general orthopaedic use.

Still, the conservative approximations used for the ASTM protocols usually make the accuracy prediction of mechanical risk less than the accuracy provided by properly used analytical methods. Using the ASTM protocols will often result in a part that is overdesigned for its application. For example, the ASTM test protocol for femoral stems requires the load on the head to be directed parallel to the axis of the stem, or the femoral canal into which the stem is placed. This loading, although conservative, is highly unrealistic. Thus the neck diameter must be made greater than necessary in order to pass the test thereby reducing the range of motion of the device. A more realistic test protocol would be useful to optimize device function in such cases.

The designer should insure that an unrealistic test does not degrade the design. If testing is required a realistic test should be performed if passing a standard test will degrade the design. When regulators require testing and a designer feels a standard test will produce failure in that test, but analysis clearly shows the design will not fail, the designer should develop a realistic test and propose this test, giving the analytical methodology and results to the regulator. With proper explanation it is likely the regulator will accept the more realistic test or may even eliminate the testing requirement.

2.4 Wear

2.4.1 Introduction

The most serious mechanical complication is wear rather than fracture or deformation of the metallic elements of a device. Examples of serious wear may be seen in Figs 2.3-2.6 which show the effects of various wear modes.

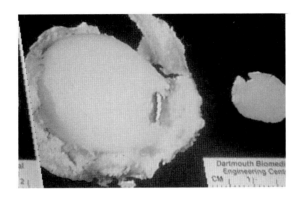

Fig. 2.3 Failed Metal-Backed Button Type Patellar Component.

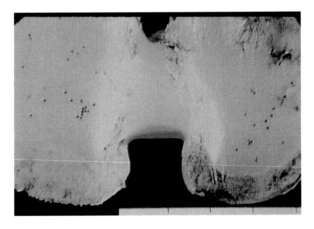

Fig. 2.4 Typical Failed PCA Bearing.

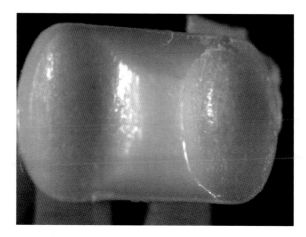

Fig. 2.5 Total Condylar Tibial Component Showing Fatigue Pits.

Polyethylene wear has received much attention due to catastrophic problems with metal-backed patellar [9, 10] and tibial prostheses [11, 12]. Such wear has been recognized by scientific investigators and clinicians as a major problem for some time [13-18].

There are concerns regarding wear in the hip [19, 20] as well as in the knee.

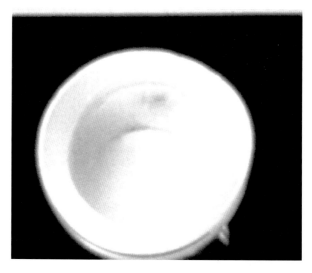

Fig. 2.6 Worn Through Acetabular Cup, 17 Year Retrieval.

Wear related problems involve wear-through, break-up, and the physiological effects of wear debris [20, 21].

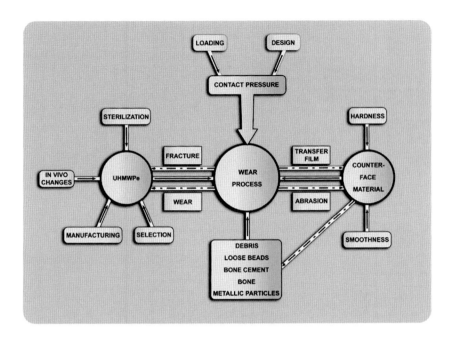

Fig. 2.7 Factors Contributing to High Wear.

Fig. 2.7 illustrates the interaction of factors affecting wear. It should be noted that the exact effect of these factors or the wear phenomena is poorly understood even in light of the large amount of literature and theories on wear. Thus, general, accurate, estimation of wear behavior is not possible and very carefully controlled and designed testing is essential in determining wear properties

To better understand the wear phenomena and what can be done to reduce wear, and its undesirable effects, one needs to examine; abrasive, adhesive, three body, and fatigue related wear; contact pressures and stresses; and the relationship between design and wear.

2.4.2 Abrasive Wear

Abrasive wear results from direct contact between the metal and plastic components. Even polished surfaces are microscopically rough. If the metal is allowed direct contact with the plastic peaks (asperities) on the metal surface will slowly gouge (abrade) away the plastic as the metal surface moves over the plastic surface, much as very fine sandpaper abrades away a wooden surface.

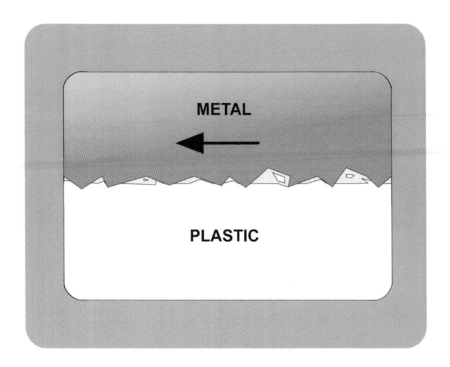

Fig. 2.8 Abrasive Wear.

The rate of abrasion is a function of the smoothness of the metal surface, the rate declining as the height of the asperities decline (the metal becomes smoother) [22].

In most machinery, bearings are in, relatively constant, unidirectional motion. When the sliding velocity is sufficient a lubricating film separates the surfaces, avoiding direct contact, and therefore abrasion. This is a hydrodynamic effect where the load is supported by a film resulting from a relative velocity between the surfaces. The parts float on this film of lubricant much as a water skier is supported by his velocity relative to the water. Under such conditions wear is negligible.

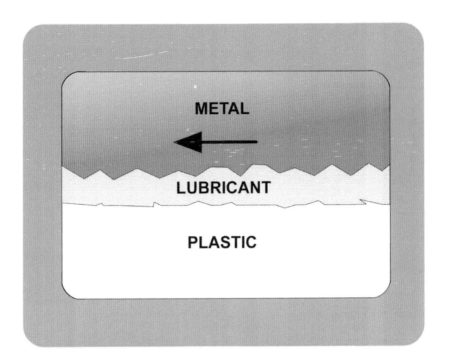

Fig. 2.9 Hydrodynamic Lubrication.

Unfortunately, human joint motion is oscillatory and therefore has substantial periods of low and zero velocity, as illustrated in Fig. 2.10, where a hydrodynamic film as shown in Fig. 2.9 cannot be sustained.

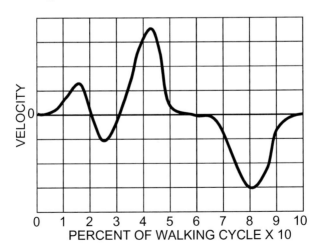

Fig. 2.10 Sliding Velocity During Walking.

In such cases one has either boundary film lubrication, where some lubrication components act to partially separate the surfaces, or dry lubrication, where there is no separating effect of the lubricant

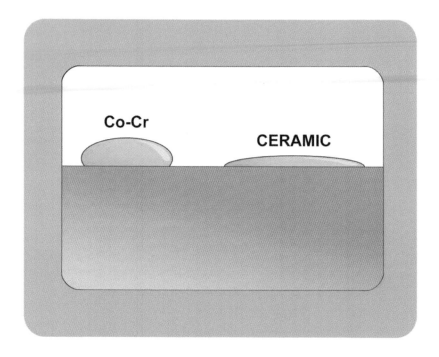

Fig. 2.11 Improved Wettability of Ceramic Surfaces.

Human joint motion is characterized by a predominance of boundary and the more destructive dry lubrication. Boundary lubrication is improved, and the period of dry lubrication is reduced, if the wettability of the surfaces is increased.

2.4.3 Adhesive Wear

This type of wear results from localized welding and tearing, rather than gouging, of the contacting surfaces.

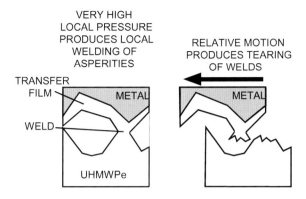

Fig. 2.12 Local Welding and Tearing of Asperities.

When opposing asperities contact each other the greatly localized nature of the contact produces such high stresses that if the two materials in contact are similar they will become welded or adherent. Translation of one with respect to the other will then produce tearing or rupture of one or both of the asperities as illustrated in Fig. 2.12.

This phenomenon is dominant after the development of a polyethylene transfer film on the Co-Cr surface of the articulating couple shown in Fig. 2.13.

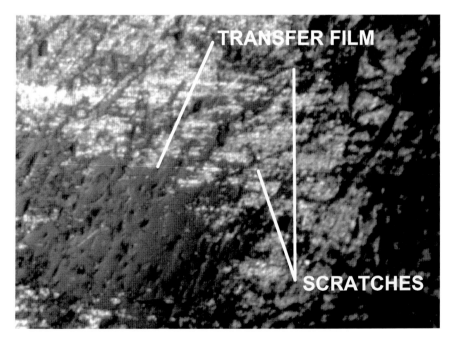

Fig. 2.13 Transfer Film on a Worn Co- Cr Femoral Head.

Just as the Co-Cr abrades the UHMWPe, the UHMWPe will also abrade the Co-Cr (albeit much more slowly). This roughened Co-Cr provides a base for the adherence of an UHMWPe film. One then has similar materials in contact, and thus the proper conditions for adhesive wear. The wear rate under these adhesive conditions is much higher than that associated with smooth surface abrasive wear as illustrated in Fig. 2.14 [23].

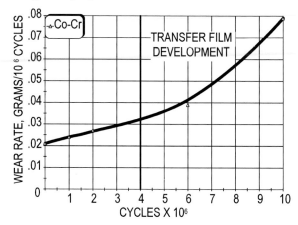

Fig. 2.14 UHMWPe Wear with 32mm Femoral Heads [23].

Such wear can apparently be minimized with ceramic- UHMWPe articulations [23].

2.4.4 Third-Body Wear

The presence of contaminants such as cement, bone debris, and loose metallic beads, as well as the wear debris of the articulating couple, also contribute to wear. This contribution is called "three-body wear".

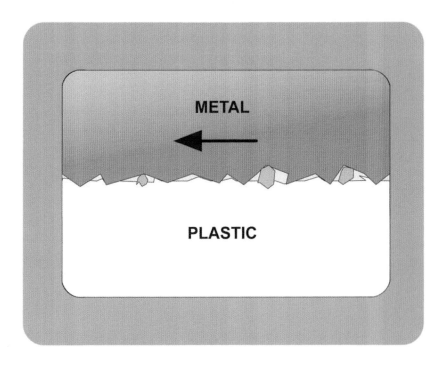

Fig. 2.15 Third-Body Wear.

Typically the harder bodies become embedded in the soft bearing as illustrated in Fig. 2.16(note: the embedded beads in Fig. 2.4). These bodies then can rapidly abrade the metal surface increasing abrasive and adhesive wear. The much harder ceramic surfaces are more resistant to the effects of such contaminants.

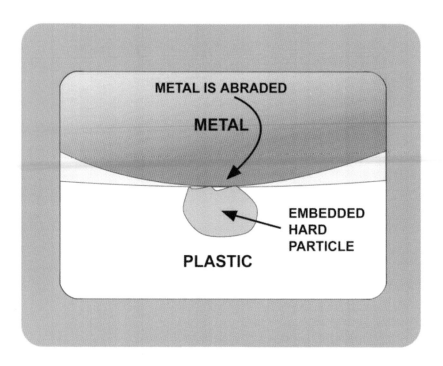

Fig. 2.16 Effect of an Embedded Hard Particle.

2.4.5 Surface Fatigue

The dominant wear (perhaps better called "fatigue failure") mode in knee replacements is fatigue related due to breakup under excessive fluctuating stress. Incongruent bodies in contact under load will deform and produce an area of contact, or a contact patch. The highest equivalent, or Von-Mises, stress σ_{eq} will be about 1mm below the surface of the UHMWPe near the center of the patch as illustrated in Fig. 2.17.

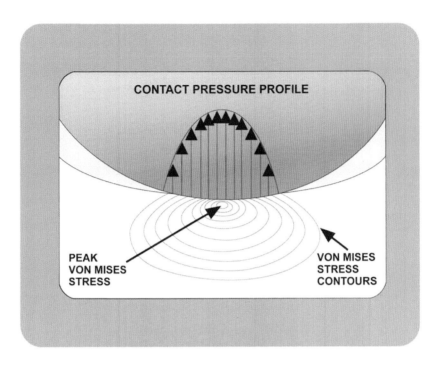

Fig. 2.17 Stress Contours for Incongruent Contact.

As the metal component slides and rolls over the surface of the weaker plastic surface the point of peak stress will move under the surfaces of the plastic as illustrated in Fig. 2.18.

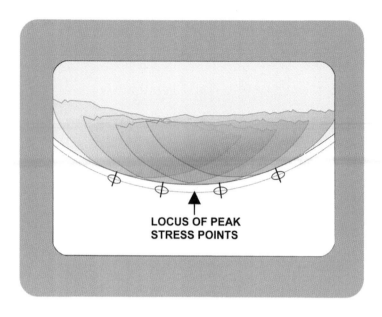

Fig. 2.18 Movement of Peak Von Mises Stress.

If the stress is high enough cracks will initiate below the surface as illustrated in Fig. 2.19.

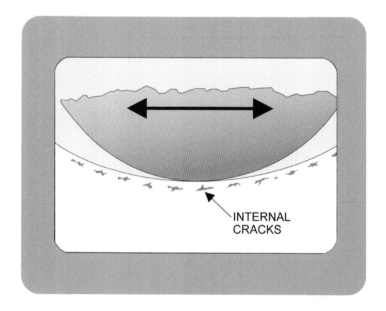

Fig. 2.19 Sub-Surface Crack Initiation.

The cracks may then coalesce to produce pitting, delamination, and by propagation through the part, catastrophic failure as illustrated if Fig. 2.20. This is a classic mode of surface failure in rolling contact [24].

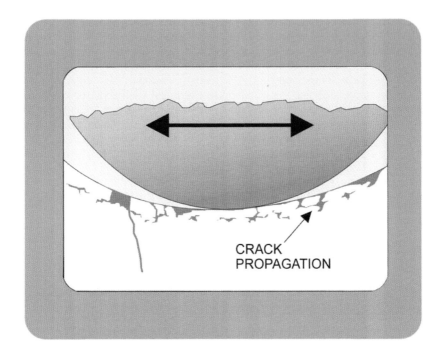

Fig. 2.20 Crack Propagation.

Such catastrophic wear is seen in Fig. 2.21.

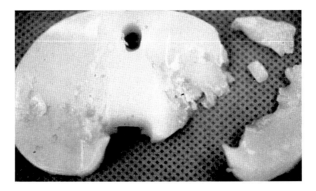

Fig. 2.21 Fatigue Failure of PCA Fixed Bearing Knee.

2.4.5.1 Contact Stress

Ordinary FEA boundary conditions cannot be used to compute incongruent contact stresses since the deformation patch is not known and thus one does not know where to apply node forces or what these forces are. Specialized software is needed which can handle incongruent contact. Such software, although generally available, is expensive and is not part of generalized mechanical CAD packages.

Fortunately, equations, sufficient for use in incongruent knee prostheses, for the computation of the contact stress of two bodies in contact were developed in the 1930's using elasticity methods [24]. The main limitation of these equations is that they do not account for the reinforcing effect of metal backed plastic components and thus tend to underestimate stresses in the linear region. On the other hand in the plastic region stress is overestimated. Still for the type of incongruent contact found in implants they are easy to use and useful since they can identify potentially safe and unsafe designs. Computations can readily be carried out by a computational program such as MathCAD.

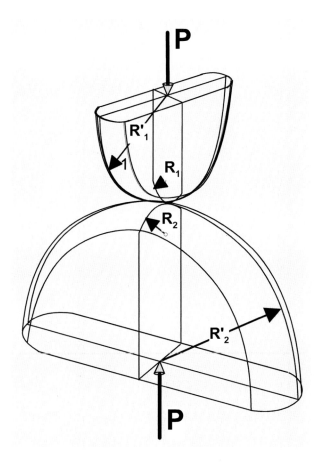

Fig. 2.22 Two Bodies in Contact.

These equations are given in [25] as well and discussed in [17]. They reduce to

$$\sigma_p = K \, (\, P \,)^{1/3} \tag{8}$$

where σ_p is the peak stress, P the applied load, and K a constant which is a function of the difference in the principal radii of curvature of the bodies at the point of contact and the stiffness of the bodies. Increased stiffness and difference in contact radii produce increased stress.

It seems clear from the typically excessive stresses found in most knee designs that most designers are either unaware of such equations, or disregard their teaching.

2.4.5.2   Analysis and Testing

a)   *Contact Pressures and Stresses*

A theoretical and experimental study of contact stress [25] demonstrates the superiority of the mobile bearing tibiofemoral articulation. Using a load of 2200N and 15° of flexion the contact stress is computed using the equations given in Refs. [24, 25]. The contact stress values were then also determined using pressure sensitive film as shown in Fig. 2.23.

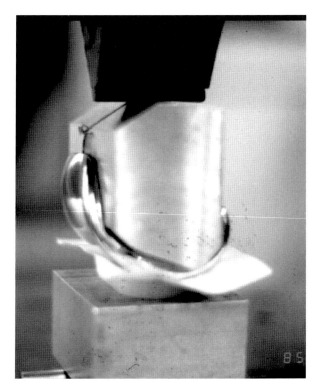

Fig. 2.23 Contact Stress Determination Using Pressure Sensitive Film.

The study tested four typical articulations as shown in Fig. 2.24. It should be noted that the "area" contact device is not fully congruent. There is a difference in radii of about 1.5%. These equations are not valid for full congruency which may be computed simply by P/A where A is a known contact area.

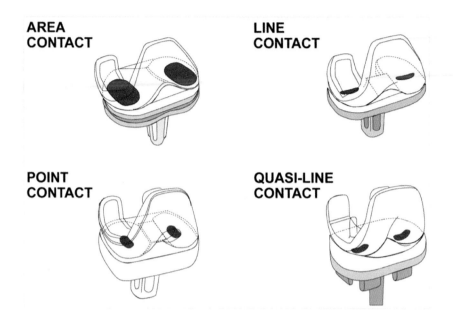

Fig. 2.24 Contact Types Evaluated.

The results for both computed and measured stresses are shown in Fig. 2.25.

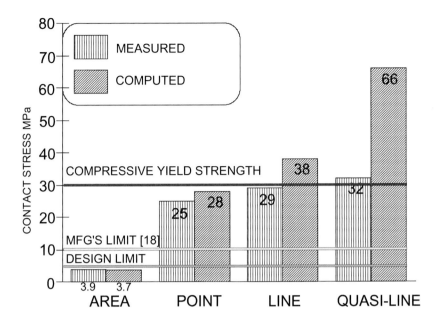

Fig. 2.25 Surface Contact Stresses for the Four Contact Types Evaluated.

It may be seen from Fig. 2.25 that at acceptable levels of stress (about 10MPa [26]), agreement of theory and experiment yields similar results.   Thus the elasticity solution is tractable at acceptable stress levels and degree of incongruity. The effect of metal backing is not significant at such incongruity and stress.

The equations appear to provide a reasonable estimate of stress in the "point" contact device. This result is, however, misleading. It is likely that the underestimation due to the metal backing is compensated by the overestimation associated with the use of elastic equations in the plastic stress range. The overestimation appears greater at the higher stress levels near the yield strength since the actual stress cannot be substantially greater than yield.

Still, there is little design value in obtaining accurate stress estimates well beyond acceptable stress levels. This elasticity method is, thus, useful for evaluating whether designs are acceptable with regard to contact stress.

Further, it may be seen that only the contact stresses in the "area" (mobile bearing) type are within reasonable limits. The other types (fixed bearings) have stresses, greatly exceeding acceptable limits, even approaching, or exceeding, the compressive yield stress of UHMWPe which is about 30MPa [25].

a)   Wear Simulator Testing
An early two million cycle simulator test showed rapid pitting of a typical incongruent fixed bearing knee, serious pitting developing within 100K cycles. There was only minor abrasive wear of the mobile bearing knee [18]. More recently [27] a new simulator was used in an effort to obtain quantitative data on knee wear. The details of the machine are shown in Figs. 26-31.

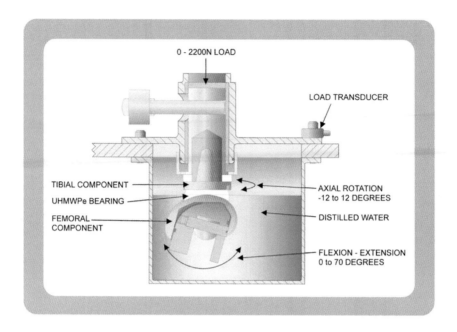

Fig. 2.26 Test Cell.

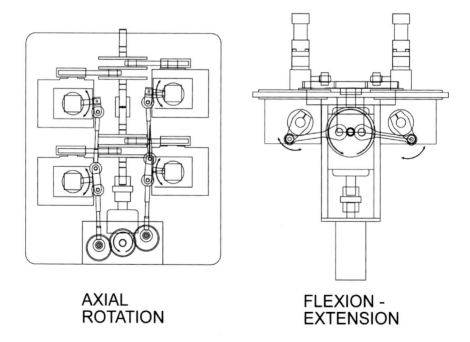

AXIAL
ROTATION

FLEXION -
EXTENSION

Fig. 2.27 Motion Schematic.

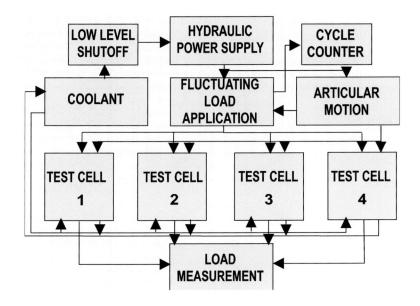

Fig. 2.28 N.J. Knee Simulator Schematic.

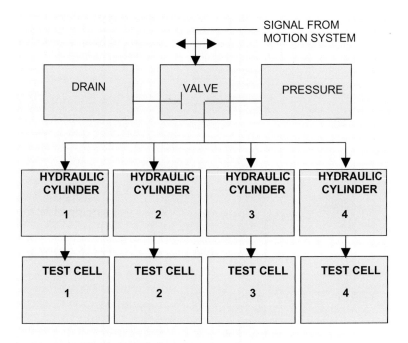

Fig. 2.29 Loading System Schematic.

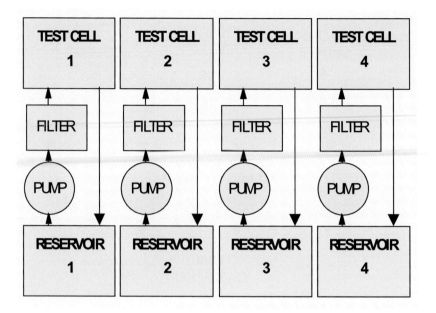

Fig. 2.30 Cooling-Lubrication System Schematic.

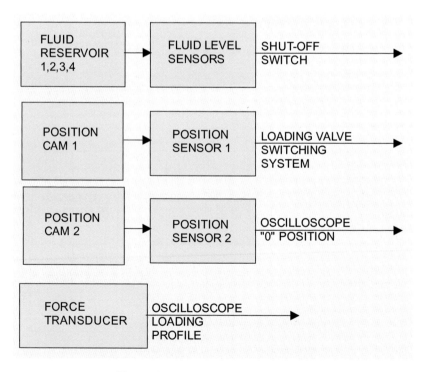

Fig. 2.31 Monitoring System Schematic.

The testing conditions were:

Motion;	0-70° Flexion-Extension
Lubricant	Distilled Water
Speed	5 Hz
Loading	0-2200N Simulated Walking

Two tests were run. A ten million cycle test, without axial rotation, of the devices of [17]; and a two million cycle test, with +/- 12° of axial rotation, of a mobile bearing [MB] and three, point contact, fixed bearing, [FB] devices. The second test was limited to 2M cycles since all the fixed bearings were worn out by that point.

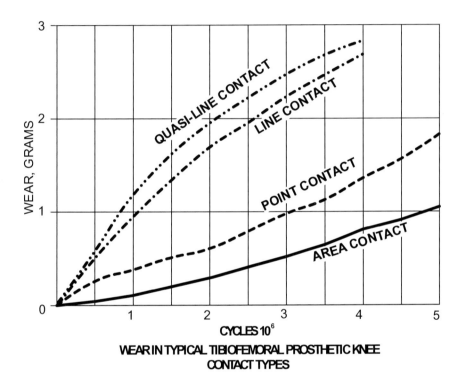

Fig. 2.32 Ten Million Cycle Test without Axial Rotation.

The wear for the first five million cycles of the 10 million cycle test are shown in Fig. 2.32 since the fixed bearing designs did not survive the entire test. The results of this test are: 1) Relative wear is consistent with the value of the contact stresses found in the study of Ref. [25], i.e. higher contact pressures produce higher wear. 2) All incongruent designs show an initial decrease in wear rate (slope of the wear curve) indicating "bedding-in" of the surfaces. The more highly incongruent designs took longer to bed-in. 3) The area contact device and the less incongruent point contact device (after an initial bedding-in) showed the expected increase in wear with time resulting from the degeneration of the Co-Cr surfaces.

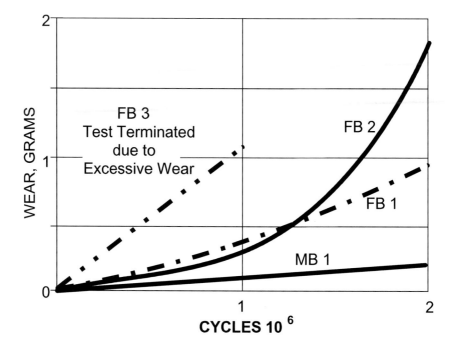

Fig. 2.33 Two Million Cycle Test with +/-12° of Axial Rotation.

The more realistic two million cycle test with axial rotation, however, showed no tendency toward bedding-in as illustrated in Fig. 2.33. No decrease in wear rate was found for any device. Thus, bedding-in is an artifact of the lack of axial rotation during simulation and does not occur to any significant degree where such rotation is present. It is, therefore, very likely bedding-in does not occur to any significant degree in vivo.

Although these tests are rather severe and thus are somewhat unrealistic, they do demonstrate the superiority of mobile bearings with regard to wear and fracture resistance.

2.4.6 Misconceptions

2.4.6.1 Bedding - In

Nevertheless, there is the common misconception that excessive contact stress known to exist in fixed bearing designs will somehow disappear as a result of some combination of deformation and "bedding - in". This process will somehow provide the congruency needed to sustain normal loads since the original design geometry clearly cannot.

As demonstrated by these tests this concept is nonsense since the complex motion of the knee means that the femoral condyles move over the surface of the tibial articulating surface and, thus, point loading occurs over a region of the tibial surface rather than at discrete points on the surface where bedding-in could occur. Therefore, for one loading cycle, deformation or wear will occur at one point and at some other point for the next loading cycle. This random motion will not produce significant bedding-in since the location and shape of femoral condylar contact continuously changes. For significant bedding-in there must be a reasonable consistency of contact region and shape.

The two year Total Condylar retrieval of Fig. 2.5 shows evidence of surface fatigue due to overloading rather than some bedding-in process.

2.4.6.2 Minimum Thickness

Another misconception is that if a tibial bearing is 6mm thick it is satisfactory with respect to contact stress. This misconception comes from a misinterpretation of Ref. [15]. This study simply indicates that as the thickness declines below 6mm the rate of stress increase becomes significantly larger than at greater thicknesses. It does not indicate that a 6mm thick component is safe. An annotated version of the data of Ref. [15] is given in Fig. 2.34. Added here are the values of compressive incongruent contact surface yielding pressure estimated from the

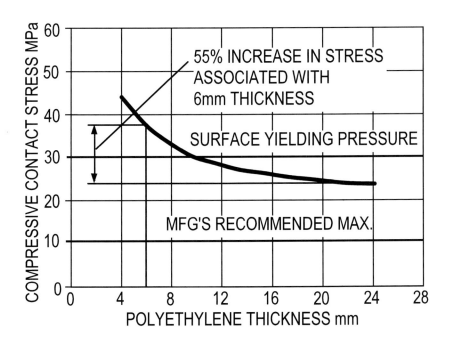

Fig. 2.34 Contact Stress as a Function of UHMWPe Thickness.

results of Ref. [25], the manufacturer's maximum recommended compressive bearing pressure for UHMWPe [26], and the increase in stress resulting from metal backing where a 6mm thick bearing is used. It may be seen that the 6mm bearing studied in Ref. [19] produces an increase in stress of more than 50%, a stress above the yield strength of the UHMWPe. At all thicknesses, however, the stress is above acceptable levels.

It should be noted this graph is associated with a particular articulation configuration studied in Ref. [15]. *More* congruent articulations have *lower* contact stress and are *less* sensitive to thickness. *Less* congruent configurations have *higher* contact stress and are *more* sensitive to thickness. Thus each design must be judged individually and cannot be judged simply on the basis of bearing thickness. No current fixed bearing designs we have studied even approach satisfactory values of contact stress.

2.4.6.3 Double Articulating Surfaces

There is a common misconception that since mobile bearing knees have two sets of articulating surfaces, which will be referred to as the "primary" femoral against tibial bearing articulation and the "secondary" tibial bearing to tibial tray articulation, the combined wear of these two surfaces will be higher than that of a fixed bearing knee with only a single primary articulating surface [28].

There are two fundamental reasons why this is invalid, at least for the LCS knee. These are:

a) Primary Wear
The wear associated with the primary articulating surface of a properly designed mobile bearing knee will be very much less than that associated with a typical fixed bearing knee. Only a mobile bearing knee has been shown to provide reasonable congruency with necessary mobility [29]. The congruency of the mobile bearing knees, such as the LCS, the ability to maintain this congruency in the presence of axial knee rotation and other knee motions, and the lack of unnecessary constraint forces resulting from unnecessary constraints, reduces contact pressures in such knees to values that are only a small fraction of those found in typical fixed bearing knees [17]. Lower pressure results in lower wear. Thus primary articulating surface wear in the LCS type knees would be expected to be much less than in a typical fixed bearing knee.

b) Secondary Wear
The wear at the secondary articulating surface is much less than at the primary articulating surface. Thus the effect of wear at the secondary articulating surface is not a major factor.

1) Consider the relative sliding distances associated with the primary and secondary articulating surfaces as shown in Fig. 2.35. It may be seen that the sliding distance associated with secondary articulation *is only a fraction of the distance associated with primary articulation.*

2) The secondary articulating surfaces are perfectly congruent for all knee motions while the primary articulating surfaces are in slightly incongruent, quasi

area, and in incongruent, quasi line at flexion angles beyond 35°. Thus wear associated with secondary articulation is expected to be only a small fraction of the wear associated with the primary articulation.

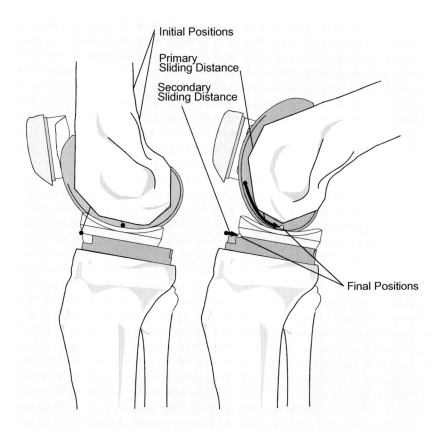

Fig. 2.35 Primary and Secondary Sliding Distances.

c) Conclusion
Since mobile bearing primary articulating surface wear is expected to be small compared to the wear associated with fixed bearing knees, and since secondary articulating surface wear is small compared to mobile bearing primary articulating surface wear, one can conclude that total mobile bearing knee wear is expected to be small compared to fixed bearing knees.

d) Clinical and Simulator Evaluation
A recent study by Collier of LCS retrievals found that back surface wear did not result in an appreciable removal of material even in those bearings of longest duration [30]. The inferior surface wear in fixed bearings is the result of micromotion and extreme stresses of the incongruent primary articulation.

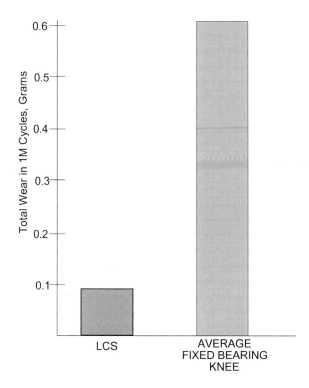

Fig. 2.36 Wear in the LCS and the Average Fixed Bearing Knee [31].

The simulator study of Ref. [31] shows total average wear of the fixed bearings tested was about six times higher than the LCS as illustrated in Fig. 2.36.

Thus these studies validate the analytical conclusion that secondary surface wear will not negate the obvious advantages of the mobile bearing concept.

e)   *Observation*
The paucity of documented bearing wear failures of the LCS knee after almost 30 years of clinical use, and the multitude of reports of fixed bearing wear failures, speaks forcefully to this issue.

2.4.7   Other Wear Related Design Considerations

2.4.7.1   Provision for Adequate Axial Rotation

It is a simple matter to produce a fully congruent design. Congruency, by itself however, is not sufficient. This is evidenced by the early Geomedic-Geometric designs which fail to provide adequate provision for axial rotation [32]. Mobility is needed along with congruity. Many later, incongruent, designs also fail to provide adequate axial rotation.

Consider a typical incongruent design as in Fig. 2.37.

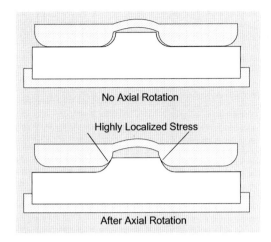

Fig. 2.37 Increased Contact Stress during Axial Rotation.

It may be seen that axial rotation can substantially change the nature of the surface contact. In properly designed mobile bearings the nature of the contact does not change as the bearing moves with the femoral component.

2.4.7.2 Provision for Abduction

Abduction of the knee occurs during the swing phase of the walking cycle, and during other normal activities. Although loads during the swing phase are relatively low they are still significant. To minimize wear the articulating surfaces must accommodate such wear. The PCA design (and the Osteonics device) is a classic case of failure to accommodate such motion.

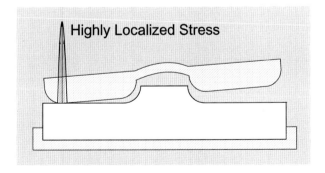

Fig. 2.38 Edge Loading During Abduction.

As illustrated in Fig. 2.38 this design, even at low loads, can produce large stresses under abduction.

Use of properly designed femoral articulating surfaces (preferably spherical) can properly accommodate abduction.

2.4.8 Summary

Abrasive wear can be reduced by smoother, and harder metallic or ceramic surfaces, and by a reduction in contact pressures.

Adhesive wear can be reduced by smoother, and harder metallic or ceramic surfaces, and by a reduction in contact pressures.

Third body wear can be reduced by harder metallic or ceramic surfaces, and by a reduction in contact pressures.

Surface fatigue wear can be reduced by a reduction in contact pressures.

Wear in incongruent knee prostheses is much higher than in hip prostheses.

Reduction in contact pressures through use of mobile bearings is the principal weapon in the fight against the degenerative effects of wear debris in knees.

Wear reduction is needed.

2.5 Biological Failure

Just as mechanical failure leads to poor function, biological failure of an artificial joint replacement can lead to significantly worse complications or even death. The most commonly encountered biological failure modes are: infection, osteolysis, progressive osteoporosis, avascular necrosis, peri-prosthetic fracture and tumor formation.

2.5.1 Infection

Septic joint replacements occur in 1-2% of cases overall [33]. The gram positive organisms of staph aureus and staph epidermides are most common and generally thought to occur at the time of initial surgery or shortly afterwards if the skin incision fails to heal in a timely fashion. Most studies prefer a delayed exchange revision approach for infected joints [34], but good success has been achieved in primary exchange techniques if the nutritional status of the patient is satisfactory and the wound heals without delay [35]. The danger of a septic joint replacement is that generalized sepsis and death can occur if the organism is virulent and fails to respond to surgical debridement and antibiotic management.

2.5.2 Osteolysis

Small (submicron) polyethylene or metallic wear particles incite an inflammatory process, whereby macrophages and giant cells, phagocytose the particles and attempt to digest them with lyzozymes and proteolytic enzymes. Unfortunately, the wear particles persist in the cytoplasm of these cells and continue to stimulate digestive enzyme production, which spills over into the surrounding bone and begins to digest this host bone. Once enough bone is lost in this osteolytic process, a cystic cavity filled with these macrophages and giant cells replaces the normal bone and begins to expand if the threshold for particle volume is exceeded. In hip replacements, the threshold for volumetric wear debris correlates with linear wear rates greater than 0.1 mm per year in an UHMWPe acetabular cup [36].

If the osteolytic cysts become too large, then fixation failure of the implant can occur, requiring revision, curettage and bone grafting of these defects to regain stability and function.

2.5.3 Progressive Osteoporosis

Disuse atrophy of the bone, also known as progressive osteoporosis occurs when the patient fails to load the bone sufficiently to maintain its strength and integrity. Regardless of the reason, such as a stroke for example, the host bone atrophies around the joint replacement and the device may loosen or the surrounding bone may fracture due to its weakened condition. Such failures are difficult to manage unless necessary loads can be applied to the bone to stimulate osteogenesis and the patient's metabolic profile can be stabilized by nutritional and hormonal support.

2.5.4 Avascular Necrosis

Vascular compromise to supporting bone causes bone cell death, known as avascular necrosis or osteonecrosis. If the region of bone is in the talus, an ankle replacement will fail due to collapse of the talar component into avascular bone [37]. In the knee, the femoral condyle or tibial plateau may develop this disorder causing collapse or loosening of the femoral or tibial component [38]. In resurfacing hip replacement, femoral head osteonecrosis can lead to femoral neck fracture and implant failure [39], which is why many surgeons prefer to avoid this procedure in favor of the more predictable stem-type hip replacement [40].

2.5.5 Peri-prosthetic Fracture

Although there is a mechanical component to fractures surrounding joint replacement implants, it is a failure of the bone that creates instability and can even be life-threatening if sufficient fat emboli compromise cardio-vascular function. These fractures must be stabilized to preserve joint function. Often, removal and revision of components are necessary in the stabilization process, combined with alternative fixation devices and immobilizing casts or braces.

2.5.6 Tumor Formation

Pseudotumors or malignant tumors can compromise a well-functioning joint arthroplasty. Pseudotumors generally form from wear debris particles that accumulate in bursal regions like the iliopsoas in the hip or the popliteal region in the knee. They can be removed surgically, while the cause for their development is addressed, namely revising the arthroplasty with more wear resistant bearings [41]. Malignant tumors are rarely associated with joint replacement, but have been reported to erode the bony fixation of implants, making them unreconstructable. Amputations or custom limb-salvage implants may be needed to provide limited function for these unfortunate patients with limited lifespan.

2.6 Conclusion

The behavior of implants in the harsh, corrosive and fluctuating load bearing environment is complex. The understanding of this behavior and the development of principles predicting such behavior are essential in the evaluation and design of orthopaedic implants.

References

[1] Harris, E.C.: Elements of Structural Engineering. Roland Donald Press, New York (1954)

[2] Ludema, K.C.: Wear. In: ASM Handbook, Friction, Lubrication, and Wear Technology, vol. 18, pp. 175–280 (1992)

[3] Amenzade, Y.A.: Theory of Elasticity. Mir, Moscow (1979)

[4] Black, J.: Biological Performance of Materials - Fundamentals of Biocompatibility. Marcel Dekker, New York (1981)

[5] Deutshman, A.D., Michels, W.J., Wilson, C.E.: Machine Design, ch. 6. Macmillan, New York (1976)

[6] Hutton, D.V.: Fundamentals of Finite Element Analysis. McGraw-Hill, New York (2004)

[7] Crowell, H.P.: Three Dimensional Finite Element Analysis of a Tibial Ankle Prosthesis. Dissertaion. New Jersey Institute of Technology (1990)

[8] Yau, S.F.: A Three-Dimensional Finite Element Stress Analysis of Interface Conditions in Porous Coated Hip Prosthesis. Dissertaion. New Jersey Institute of Technology (1991)

[9] Stulberg, S.D., et al.: Failure mechanisms of metal-backed patellar components. Clinical Orthopaedics and Related Research 236, 88–105 (1988)

[10] Bourne, R.B., et al.: Metal-backed total knee replacement patellar components: a major problem for the future. In: Paper No. 315 Presented at the 58th Annual Meeting of the AAOS (1990)

[11] Jones, S.M.G., et al.: Polyethylene wear in uncemented knee replacements. Journal of Bone and Joint Surgery[Br] 74B(1), 18–22 (1992)

[12] Engh, G.A., Dwyer, K.A., Hannes, C.K.: Polyethylene wear of metal-backed tibial components in total and unicompartmental knee prostheses. Journal of Bone and Joint Surgery [Br] 74B(1), 9–17 (1992)

[13] Rose, R.M., Goldfarb, E.V., Ellis, E., Crugnola, A.M.: On pressure dependence of the wear of ultra high molecular weight polyethylene. Wear 92, 99–111 (1983)

[14] Bartel, D.L., et al.: Performance of the tibial component of the total knee replacement. Journal of Bone and Joint Surgery (Am) 64A, 1026 (1982)

[15] Bartel, D.L., Bicknell, V.L., Wright, T.M.: The effect of conformity, thickness and material on stresses in ultra-high molecular weight polyethylene components for total joint replacement. Journal of Bone and Joint Surgery (Am) 68A, 1041 (1986)

[16] Ravell, P.A., et al.: The production and biology of polyethylene wear debris. Archives of Orthopaedic and Traumatic Surgery 91, 167–181 (1997)

[17] Pappas, M.J., Makris, G., Buechel, F.F.: Evaluation of contact stress in metal plastic knee replacements. In: Pizzoferrato, A., et al. (eds.) Biomaterials and Clinical Applications, pp. 259–264. Elsevier, Amsterdam (1997); Clemson SC:101

[18] Pappas, M.J., Buechel, F.F.: New Jersey knee simulator. In: Proceedings of the Eleventh International Biomaterials Symposium held at Clemson SC, vol. 101 (1979)

[19] Bartell, D.L., Wright, T.M., Edwards, D.L.: The effect of metal backing on stresses in polyethylene acetabular components. In: The Hip: Proceedings of Hip Society, vol. 229, CV Mosby, St. Louis (1983)

[20] Willert, H.G., Semlitsh, M.: Reaction of the articular capsule to wear products of artificial joint prostheses. Journal of Biomedical Materials Research 11, 134–164 (1977)

[21] Gelante, J.O., et al.: The Biological Effects of Implant Materials. Journal Of Orthopaedic Research 9, 760–775 (1991)

[22] Dowson, D., et al.: Influence of counterface topography on the wear ofUHMWPE under wet and dry condifions. In: Lee, H.L. (ed.) The Proceedings of the American Chemical Society, Polymer Wear and tis Control. ACS Symp. Ser., vol. 287, pp. 171–187 (1985)

[23] Pappas, M.J., et al.: Comparison of Wear Of UHMWPe Cups Articulating With Co Cr and TiN Coated Femoral Heads. Transactions of the Society of Biomaterials XIII, 36 (1990)

[24] Seely, F.B., Smith, J.O.: Advanced Mechanics of Materials, ch.14. Wiley and Sons, New York (1958)

[25] Pappas, M.J., Makris, G., Buechel, F.F.: Contact stresses in metal plastic total knee replacements: A theoretical and experimental study. Biomedical Engineering Technical Report. Biomedical Engineering Trust, South Orange NJ (1986)

[26] Hostalen, G.U.R.: Hoechst Aktiengesellschaft, Verkauf Kunstoffe, 6230 Frankfurt am Main 80, 22 (1982)

[27] Pappas, M.J., Makris, G., Buechel, F.F.: Wear in prosthetic knee joints. In: Scientific Exhibit, 59th Annual Meeting of the AAOS, Washington, DC (1992)

[28] Pappas, M.J.: LCS White Paper #1, Two Articulating Surface Wear of UHMWPe Bearings. Biomedical Engineering Trust, Trust South Orange NJ (1994)

[29] Pappas, M.J., Buechel, F.F.: N.J. Integrated Knee Replacement System: Rationale and Review of 193 Cases. Biomedical Engineering Technical Report. Biomedical Engineering, Trust South Orange NJ (1984)

[30] Collier, J.P., Williams, I.R., Mayor, M.B.: Retrieval Analysis of Mobile Bearing Prosthetic Knee Devices. In: Hamelynck, K.J., Stiehl, J.B. (eds.) LCS Mobile Bearing Knee Arthroplasty: 25 Years of Worldwide Experience, pp. 74–80. Springer, Heidelberg (2002)

[31] Pappas, M.J., Makris, G., Buechel, F.F.: Wear in Prosthetic Knee Joints. In: Scientific Exhibit, 59th Annual Meeting of the AAOS, Washington, DC (1992)

[32] Riley, D., et al.: Long Term Results of Geomedic Total Knee Replacement. JBJS 66A, 734 (1984)

[33] Buechel, F.F.: The Infected Total Knee Arthroplasty: Just When You Thought It Was Over. J. Arthroplasty 19(4(suppl. 1)), 51–56 (2004)

[34] Moyad, T.F., Thornhill, T., Estok, D.: Evaluation and Management of the Infected Total Hip and Knee. Orthopaedics 31(6), 581–588 (2008)

[35] Buechel, F.F., et al.: Primary Exchange Revision Arthroplasty for Infected Total Knee Replacement: A Long Term Study. Am. Journal of Orthop. XXXIII, 4 (2004)

[36] Hozak, W.J., Orozco, F.: Osteolysis and Total Hip Replacement. Medscape, http://cme.medscae.com/vioewarticle/420395 (accessed August 29, 2009)

[37] Buechel, F.F.: Osteolysis After Total Ankle Replacement. In: Presented at the 35th Annual Orthopaedic Surgery & Trauma Society Meeting. Bonaire, Netherlands Antilles (2009)

[38] Buechel, F.F., et al.: Twenty-year evaluation of meniscal bearing and rotating platform knee replacements. Clin. Orthop. 388, 41–50 (2001)

[39] Shimmin, A.J., Back, D.: Femoral Neck Fractures Following Birmingham Hip Resurfacing: A National Review of 50 Cases. JBJS Br. 87B(4), 463–464 (2002)

[40] Garbuz, D.S.: Metal on Metal Hip Resurfacing vs Large Diameter Hip Arthroplasty. In: Hip Society. The John Charnley Award (2009)

[41] Pandit, H., et al.: Pseudotumors Associated with Metal-on-Metal Hip Resurfacing. JBJS Br. 90B, 847–851 (2008)

Chapter 3
The Design Process

Abstract. This chapter describes the procedure that should be used for the design of orthopaedic devices. The design of such devices is controlled by regulatory authories in most countries, such as by the FDA GMP requirements and in the EU by EU Directive MDD 93/42/EC. Except for minor design changes design must be carried out following a detailed design plan with the activities associated with the plan well documented. The design process usually begins when a design opportuinty is identified. After feasibility is determined a design plan is formulated with inputs from reglatory affairs and patent expertise. Design requirements are extablished and usually, at least one, preliminary design developed and evaluated. Final design can then be developed through a feed-back process of redesign and reevaluation. The Final design must then be verified through appropriate analysis and testing. The design and associated manufacturing capability must be then validated before release for producion. This process must be documented in the Design History Files.

Definitions

- *Device,* finished product; an orthopaedic implant introduced by surgically penetrating the skin or mucosa of the body with the intention that it remain within the body following surgery.
- *Device Instrument*, instrument used during surgical procedure to implant a device.
- *Humanitarian Use Device, (HUD),* a medical device that, due to the fact that its use applies to a very limited population, may have a limited target population. HUD's distributed in the United States must meet the definitions and be handled in compliance with the provisions of 21 CFR 814.
- *Patient Adapted Device, (PAD),* Product manufactured to specification for distribution with modification or customization, to fit a patient's specific anatomy. The PAD devices that are distributed within the United States must be cleared under the 510 (k) or PMA regulations. The PAD devices that are distributed within the European Union (EU) must be

classified and CE marked the same as non-custom devices (Standard Product).

- *Trial,* Mock implant(s) used during the surgery for the purpose of checking the fit, and preliminary function tests.
- *Technical File,* This file should hold or reference the technical documentation (documents and records) that demonstrate that the family of products conform to the requirements of the EC Directive (MDD 93/42 EC). This file should be readily accessible for review by the Competent Authority. There should be one Technical File per family.
- *Design History File, (DHF),* This file should hold information on all design, design modification, validation and verification processes. This file should be readily accessible for review by the Competent Authority. There should be one DHF per family.
- *Design Committee,* representatives of Engineering, Manufacturing, QA, Medical Director, Marketing, Sales and Regulatory Affairs.
- *Evaluation,* Design Review and when applicable, other verification/ validation of the Design.
- *Engineering Model,* a model used to obtain information and data used for design purposes.
- *Design Requirement (Design Input),* the physical and performance requirements of the product that are used for its design.
- *Design Output,* the results of a design effort, the added value. At each stage of the design there should be an output that must be reviewed against the input. The *finished design output* should be the documents of the Device Master Record, i.e. the specifications, drawings, process procedures and work instruction, packaging specifications, labeling, and QA inspection procedures.
- *Design Documentation (Design Transfer),* the process of converting the design documents into the production documents that should be used for manufacture.
- *Verification,* the analysis and testing required during design development to verify conformance to the design input or specifications.
- *Validation,* the testing of the design and manufacturing process of the production design and the production manufacturing processes to validate conformance to the design input or specifications.
- *Post market Surveillance and Vigilance,* the collection and analysis of data on the performance and problems with the production design in the field.

3.1 Introduction

The manufacture of joint replacement implants and instruments is a complex process that is, in almost all countries, overseen by some official agency to guarantee adherence to strict quality standards. In the United States manufacturers must adhere to the FDA Good Manufacturing Practices (GMP) regulations [1] and in the EU countries to an International Standard Organization protocol, such as ISO 13485 and EU Directive MDD 93/42/EC [2, 3]. These manufacturing standards are enforced by periodic inspections and enforcement actions where needed.

The application and enforcement of these regulations is, however, a relatively recent event, even though they have been in place for at least two decades. As a result most of the earlier, and even some existing designs are not a product of a formal, well controlled, design procedure. They, thus, often contain important design defects.

Good design is the key to producing a quality product. The design process should ensure that the design requirements (Design Input) are understood and documented; the design should be continuously reviewed to ensure that the design output matches the design input; and that the design is thoroughly verified and validated before the design is released for production. The resulting final product must meet the requirements for the design, meet all of the design specifications for form and performance, and be introduced in a manner that is in compliance with applicable regulations (Design Input). The device must also be validated after initial production to insure that these requirements are met and will continue to be met.

Good design, unfortunately, cannot be based entirely on adherence to regulations. It must also be based on sound engineering methods and principles and the applications of such methods and principles by talented, creative designers with a high state of knowledge of the science and practice of orthopaedic implants and instrumentation. Good design involves an understanding and input from several disciplines such as Engineering, Manufacturing, QA, Medical Director, Marketing, Sales and Regulatory Affairs.

3.2 Procedure

Product design is an iterative process that demands flexibility and the ability to change the design, design inputs and design requirements. The procedure given here is intended to provide a template for guiding the design process. As such, different projects should have different requirements and all parts of this procedure may not fit every project. This should be continually assessed during the project using formal, documented, design reviews. All new designs or significant changes to existing designs should be managed under such a procedure.

It should be noted that almost all design is actually redesign of some existing product. Most design is design refinement or correction. Thus, the difference between a "new" design and a design refinement is quite subjective. Generally a good way to differentiate is interchangeability. If a design consists of components that are entirely interchangeable with an earlier design then it can be considered a design refinement. Otherwise it can be considered a new design.

An important part of this procedure is documentation of the various stages of the design process. It is necessary for all personnel involved in the design process to recognize that each step in the process should be adequately documented and retained in a Design History File (DHF) which should contain all documents and records of the design project plan and all design reviews.

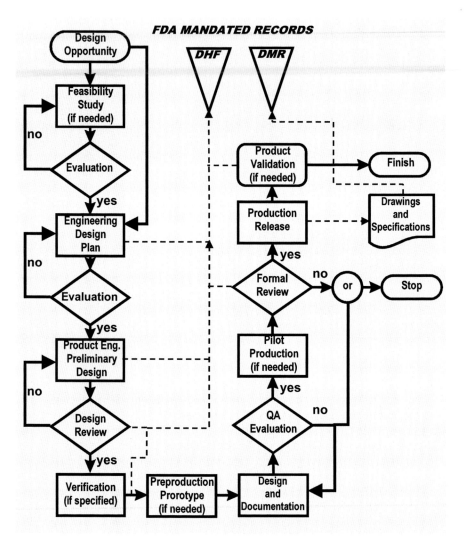

Fig. 3.1 Design Process Flowchart.

The process is illustrated in the flowchart of Fig. 3.1. It should be noted that after review and evaluation, or even during the design and testing phases the need for changes to the design, design plan or other processes may become apparent.

Thus it is expected that this iterative process may involve several, if not many, loops within the overall process.

Not all changes to an existing product are substantial enough to require formal design control. Examples are minor labeling changes and improvements to a device that do not modify its clinical performance or Indications/Contraindications, Such minor changes are to be handled using a formal Data, Document and Change Control Procedure. Changes to released documents that have been previously approved should be made using such a procedure, as well as being subject to the necessary reviews. Based on the degree of change, each previously released design or document may be subject to reevaluation by a formal "Design Committee" according to this procedure. Significant changes may require the designation of a new device design.

3.2.1 Design Opportunity

Generally management recognizes, or has brought to its attention, a design opportunity for a new product or for a design modification. Such an opportunity may arise from the desire to exploit a new scientific discovery, the need to introduce a new system to compete with one introduced by a competitor, or simply to correct some design problem or provide a design improvement.

3.2.2 Feasibility Study

If management determines it is needed, it may commission a feasibility study. A copy of this study should be retained in the DHF. Feasibility studies can be quite complex involving design concept development, manufacturability, patent considerations, regulations, finance, marketing and medical considerations. They may also be quite simple and limited to a single consideration.

3.2.2.1 Evaluation

Where a feasibility study is developed, management evaluates the study to determine whether to proceed with the design or to investigate related design opportunities. This decision should be recorded in the DHF.

3.2.3 Engineering Design Plan

If the decision to proceed with the project is made by management the Director of Engineering designates a Project Manager who devises and monitors a formal "Design Plan" outlining the processes of design, and designating who should be responsible for each phase of the design process, including the documenting of the design requirements. This plan should include an initial chronological developmental strategy listing milestones for the project, as well as specific requirements for assessing those milestones in order for the project to progress. As much as is possible, pass/fail criteria for each milestone should be developed at this stage. The plan is initiated after approval by the management after review and approval by a Design Committee. The Design Committee normally consists of representatives of Engineering, Manufacturing, QA, Medical Director, Marketing, Sales and Regulatory Affairs.

The Design Plan must include periodic review and approval by the Design Committee that evaluates its progress and the resulting design output. Should changes in the Plan or Input be required or desired they must be changed by a formal Change Order Procedure. As the project progresses, design outputs, in the form of data from testing or validations, should be reviewed by the Committee to ensure that Design Inputs and Design Requirements are being met.

3.2.3.1 Regulatory Affairs

As early as possible in the design process, Regulatory Affairs should provide an assessment of the U.S. and European Union regulatory requirements for introduction of all new/revised devices. This should include determining whether the new/revised device requires a PMA/PMA Supplement, Humanitarian Use Device (HUD), 510(k) pre-market notification, IDE, or clinical trial and related approvals required by the FDA or Notified Bodies, prior to its introduction into commerce. No finished revised/new devices should be distributed commercially or for clinical investigation anywhere in the United States or in the European Union unless the requirements stipulated by Regulatory Affairs, the FDA and Notified Body (as applicable) have been met.

3.2.3.2 HUD

If it is determined by Regulatory Affairs that a new/revised device qualifies as a humanitarian-use device (HUD), a Humanitarian Use Exemption (HUE) should be filed with FDA and the device may be shipped in the USA as directed in the HUE approved by the FDA.

3.2.3.3 Consultation with Regulatory Bodies

As needed, Regulatory Affairs should consult with the FDA or Notified Bodies to determine the regulatory requirements for introducing the new/revised device and then include documentation of the recommendations and/or requirements in the DHF.

3.2.3.4 Patents

Novel and useful designs may be protected by one or more patents. Prior to the full development of a new design it is essential to determine its patent status at an early stage. One should determine:

a)   If the design appears patentable and
b)   If the design infringes any active, valid patents.

The claims of a patent prevent anyone other than the patent holder, or an assignee, from using, making, or selling any device or process reading on the claims of a patent. Thus, if a new design is patentable, a patent can be useful in preventing a competitor from using the design (invention). Conversely if the new design, even if it is patentable, infringes another patent, one can be prevented from using the new design. It is clear, therefore, that an understanding of the patent status of a new design be developed early to avoid potential infringement problems. Legal costs defending against infringement can be extremely high and the cost of damages for infringement even higher.

It should also be noted that obtaining a patent can be expensive. Once a preliminary design is developed, however, one can at minimal expense, file a provisional patent describing the invention. Such a description is often needed, in any event, as part of the design review process. One then has a year to submit the formal patent draft. The design is protected from the date of submission of the provisional patent. Such early submission is important since in the event of another submission on the same invention the earlier submission date establishes the inventor of record. The inventor of record is no longer established by the first to invent. It is now the first to submit.

The time between the submission of the provisional draft and the formal draft may be used to further develop the design and, more importantly, to determine if the design is worth the expense associated with obtaining and enforcing a patent. Typically, an implant invention is worth protecting but, an instrument patent is not. Every situation is, however, relatively unique and one normally makes a decision on obtaining patent protection based on the facts of each particular case.

In summary, patent consideration should be a significant part of most formal design plans.

3.2.3.5 Design Inputs

The Product Manager should initiate a Design History File by documenting the design inputs and reviewing them with the design committee to assess whether they are appropriate or require modification. Design Inputs can take many forms. Some examples of appropriate inputs are:

- Indications/Contraindications/User interfaces
- Performance/Physical/Mechanical characteristics
- Safety risk/benefit ratio requirements
    - Bio-compatibility requirements
    - Clinical requirements
    - Packaging/Labeling requirements
    - Regulatory requirements
    - Manufacturing requirements
    - Physical loading requirements
    - Motion requirements
    - Intended use of the device
    - Measurements and measuring instruments to be used

- Sterility requirements
- Lifetime of the device

In addition one should consider the following joint implant system criteria:

a) Medical and Engineering Criteria

- Material and wear product compatibility
- Adequate mechanical strength
- Minimization of the joint reaction forces
- Minimization of fixation interface tension
- Avoidance of fixation interface shear
- Uniformity of interface compression
- Duplication of anatomical function
- Adequate fit for the patient population
- Manufacturability
- Inventory costs

b) Medical and Surgical Criteria

- Treatment of a broad variety of pathologies
- Maximal preoperative options
- Maximal intraoperative options
- Maximal postoperative options in case of failure
- Salvagability
- Tolerance for misalignment
- Ease of implantation

3.2.3.6 Verification

Verification of the design should be performed at designated phases of the design process, to verify that the design output is consistent with the required input, using methods appropriate to the design as determined by the Design Committee and defined in the Design Plan. These methods may include:

- Determination of motion;
- Stress analysis;
- Simulator testing for loading and wear;
- Manufacture and testing of prototypes;
- Testing of materials;
- Biocompatibility studies;
- Comparison of the proposed design to similar approved devices on the market, including any clinical investigations;
- Risk Analysis using Failure Mode and Effects Analysis (FMEA). or other methods;
- Computer Generated Modeling.
- Assessments by independent experts

3.2.3.7 Validation

When required to assess design inputs, validations should be performed. The specific requirements for each validation should necessarily be different each time one is to be done, however, the requirements for the validation should be established in a written protocol which should then be reviewed by the Design Committee prior to performing the validation testing. In general, the protocol should include a clearly defined purpose, test/evaluation methodologies, end-points wherein the data should be assessed and the criteria to be used for accepting or rejecting its generated results.

3.2.3.8 Personnel

The Design Plan must identify specific individuals from the Design Committee who are to be involved in the design process, their assigned activities, and how these groups are to interface with each other to provide input into the design and development process. Members of the Design Committee should be assigned to establish the design input requirements and the type(s) of design output data and/or validations and verifications that the Committee requires to meet these input requirements.   To the extent possible, the Committee should establish whether each of these requirements must be reviewed and approved by the entire Committee or only by designated members and when such reviews should take place; recognizing that as the project progresses, the delegation of reviews and approvals may change based on output data. Design reviews should take place at least once per quarter, and more often as designated by the Design Committee.

The success of a design is almost entirely the result of the actions of the Design Committee personnel. Thus, it is essential that the committee be composed of highly skillful, analytical, open minded, objective and creative individuals.

For new or revised devices that represent significant changes from existing devices, the opinion of a Medical Monitor should be included as part of the Committee's review of input and output requirements that have clinical implications.

3.2.3.9 Evaluation

The Design Committee should review the Design Requirements (Design Input), including any information gathered from Post Market Surveillance and Vigilance to ensure its accuracy.

Design Reviews should be performed frequently enough to ensure that project milestones and dates are being adhered to or appropriately modified. These reviews normally are accomplished by scheduling meetings of the Design Committee and outside experts, as needed, or by having the members of the Design Committee review and approve reports or data as they are generated. In either case, the results of the review and approvals to proceed with the project should be documented in the DHF. The group reviewing the final production design should consist of the Design Committee and at least one independent expert of the device involved.

3.2.4   Preliminary Design

3.2.4.1   Design Development

Engineering first develops a preliminary design or preliminary design alternatives. Documents defining these designs should comprise the "Device Master Record" (DMR). These should include:

- New or modified drawing(s) of device
- New or modified drawing(s) of Instruments and Trials
- New or modified Material and Manufacturing instructions, device history records and inspection instructions and specifications
- New or modified Labeling specifications.
- New or modified X-ray template of the device

This phase may involve the development of one or more design concepts and the development of information obtained from engineering analysis, manufacture and test of engineering models and evaluation and testing of materials.

3.2.4.2   Review

The design committee should review the preliminary design(s) for manufacturability, conformance to all regulations and satisfaction of the design inputs.

3.2.4.3   Verification

The verification (if needed) specified in the design plan is now performed and reviewed.

3.2.4.4   Preproduction Prototypes

Pre-production prototypes should be manufactured when and as specified by the Design Plan. The prototypes should be evaluated, using appropriate verification and validation methods. In most cases, prototype devices may not be distributed to any surgeon or surgical site in the United States for use in human subjects unless approved by the Director of Regulatory Affairs. In the case of class III implants such approvals are generally part of an approved IDE study, patient-specific custom device waiver, humanitarian-use exemption, compassionate-use waiver, 510(k) approval or PMA/PMA supplement.

All documents associated with prototypes should be clearly marked with the word "PROTOTYPE". Any such documents should only be used for the manufacture or evaluation of the prototypes. These are preliminary documents and may be changed only with the approval of the Project Manager but without resorting to the formal change procedure. These documents may be based on released documents where the prototype is used to evaluate proposed changes to released parts or devices.

3.2.5 Production Design

Using the information acquired during the preliminary design process, as well as an input from the Design Committee and, perhaps, independent experts, Engineering should develop a design suitable for production and sale and associated supporting documentation.

3.2.5.1 QA Review

QA should review the device to assess its suitability for intended use and safety.

3.2.5.2 Regulatory Actions

Regulatory Affairs, should undertake activities required to obtain the necessary FDA approval (or other regulatory approvals, including CE marking), for the new/revised device. Regulatory Affairs should also document that the device continues to meet its established design criteria as well as those submitted to the pertinent regulatory agencies or otherwise ensure that appropriate documentation and validations describing and substantiating any changes from the submitted design are obtained. Regulatory approvals, as pertinent, should be obtained for any significant modifications to submitted designs for devices.

3.2.5.3 Pilot Production

There should be a "Pilot Production Run" (PPR) of the device, if specified in the Design Plan, to test and evaluate the producibility of the design, design and production documentation, the production capability and methods and to produce initial production implants and instruments for verification and validation. Results of this PPR, including manufacturing data, and verification and validation studies should be provided to the Design Committee for review and approval.

The design and production documentation associated with the device undergoing pilot production should be stamped with the words "PILOT PRODUCTION". The documents should be complete and released for pilot production prior to the start of the run and should be used during all phases to allow the evaluation of these documents under production conditions. Any such documents should only be used for the manufacture or evaluation of the pilot production units or manufacturing capability. These are preliminary documents and may be changed only with the approval of the Project Manager but without resorting to a formal procedure. These documents may be based on released documents where the pilot production is used to evaluate proposed changes to released parts or devices.

3.2.5.4 Document Changes

Other than changes to the Design Plan, which may only be altered by the formal change procedure, changes to documents occurring during the development process should be the sole responsibility of the group preparing the documents.

Copies of all versions of the documents generated during the development process should however, be dated and stored and documented in the DHF.

3.2.5.5 Formal Review

Before being released, there should be a full and formal review of all the design documents. Engineering is responsible for creating and maintaining the (DHF). Regulatory Affairs is responsible for ensuring that finished devices are not distributed in the U.S. or other countries unless required regulatory approvals have been achieved.

If the device is to be distributed within the EU, the final formal Design Review should ensure that all the essential requirements of MDD 93/42/EC are met. If the new device is to be part of a family that is CE marked, then the relevant Technical File must be amended, and a new Declaration of Conformity drawn up to include the new device.

If the device is to be distributed within the US, the final formal Design Review should ensure that it is in accordance with FDA regulations. That is, the Design Review should ensure that either a 510(k) or PMA approval is obtained if needed prior to device distribution. If neither a 510(k) nor PMA approval is needed, the rationale for that conclusion should be documented.

3.2.6 Production Release

Once management and engineering are satisfied the design is complete, verified and validated the design and associated documents are released for production and sale of the design.

3.2.6.1 DMR

The design drawings, manufacturing instructions, device history records, inspection instructions, specifications and labels are released in accordance with a formal Document Release and Change procedure. A Device Master Record (DMR) should be created for those documents.

3.2.6.2 Catalog Numbers

Marketing/Sales should create catalog numbers for the designs. Marketing should maintain a master list of catalog numbers along with their respective descriptions. These catalog numbers should be referenced in the DMR.

3.2.6.3 Validation

Orthopaedic implants are designed to work in a living human being. Thus, in many cases validation may be primarily clinical in nature and thus validation should continue after production and sale is initiated. Class III devices will normally be validated by a formal, FDA monitored, clinical trial. Class II devices are normally validated by information gathered from a formal, documented procedure for "Post Market Surveillance and Vigilance" and by clinical evaluation performed by the Medical Director. Further, where specified in the Design Plan, product from the PPR and initial production runs may also be used for validation studies.

3.2.7   Design Records

These records may include all or part of the following)

3.2.7.1   Design History File (DHR);

Which may include the:

- Design Plan;
- Design Input:
- Design Review(s);
- Verification results;
- Design Transfer Review;
- Validation results;
- Risk Analysis;
- Regulatory approvals (as applicable)
- Draft versions of documents in the DMR
- Results from any Post market Surveillance or Vigilance.
- Clinical study data (as applicable)

3.2.7.2   Device Master Record (DMR);

Which may include the:

- Drawings;
- Specifications;
- Labels;
- Work Instructions;
- Inspection procedures.

3.2.7.3   Technical File

Which may include the:

- General Description;
- Essential Requirements Checklist;
- Device Master Record (DMR);
- Labeling;
- Design History File (DHR);
- Post Market Surveillance;

- Risk Analysis;
- Clinical Studies.

References

[1]   FDA GMP Manual (820.30)
[2]   INTERNATIONAL STANDARD ISO13485 (4.4), Medical Devices – Quality management systems – Requirements for regulatory purposes, 2nd edn. (July 15, 2003)
[3]   EC Directive MDD 93/42/EC

Chapter 4
The Ankle

Abstract. This chapter describes the anatomy, pathology of the ankle and ankle replacements developed to treat pathological ankles. The history of three generations of ankle replacement designs, their evaluation in light of the material in Chapters 1 and 2 and the clinical performance of these designs are presented. The first and second generations had little success, except for the mobile bearing devices which were not available in the USA. This produced, in the United States, the incorrect perception that fusion was preferable to replacement. Unfortunately the FDA required a well controlled clinical trial for approval of a mobile bearing ankle device inhibiting the use of such devices in the USA until recently. Also presented is the design of a third generation ankle using the principles of the first three chapters. The design process of Chapter 3 was used for the development of an improved version of the LCS ankle. The B-P ankle replacement is the result. It is a mobile bearing device using ceramic coated titanium alloy for its metallic components. Early results were quite good. Unfortunately a major problem developed in long term use. Even though the wear in these devices is very low, this wear, nevertheless, produced destructive osteolytic cysts. This is a problem common to all current replacements. Perhaps improvement in manufacturing and/or materials can overcome this problem, but clearly more work and time is needed before a reliable, long term, ankle replacement becomes available.

4.1 Anatomy

The complex known as the ankle joint consists of the tibia, fibula and talus (Fig. 4.1) articulating to accommodate mainly dorsiflexion and plantarflexion and to a limited degree inversion-eversion and axial rotation.

4.1.1 Ligamentous Structures

Laterally, the ankle is stabilized by the anterior talofibular ligament (ATFL), the calcaneofibular ligament (CFL) and the posterior talofibular ligament (PTFL).
Medially, the ankle is stabilized by the deltoid ligament (Fig. 4.2).

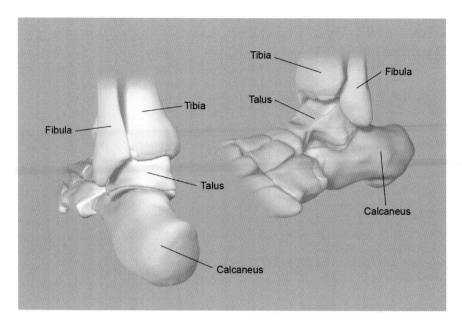

Fig. 4.1 Bones of the ankle.

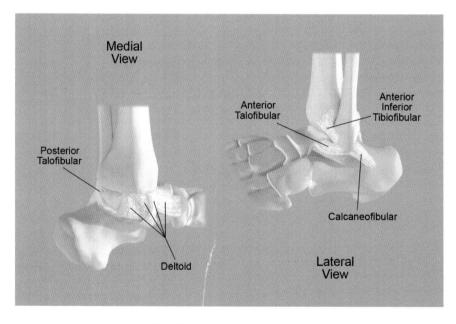

Fig. 4.2 Ligaments of the Ankle.

A shallow-sulcus is in the central surface of the talus demarcating the medial
and lateral colliculi which reside symmetrically in the ankle mortise created by the
tibiofibular articulation.

4.1.2 Musculature

The muscles of dorsiflexion in the ankle from medial to lateral include the anterior
tibialis, the extensor hallucis longus (EHL), the extensor digitorum communis and
the peroneus tertius. The muscles of plantarflexion include the gastroc-soleus
complex ending in the Achilles tendon, the flexor hallucis and to a lesser extent
the posterior tibialis, which also serves as the main muscle of inversion of the
midfoot and hindfoot. The muscles of eversion include the peroneus longus and
peroneus brevis.

The ankle tendons are shown in Fig.4.3.

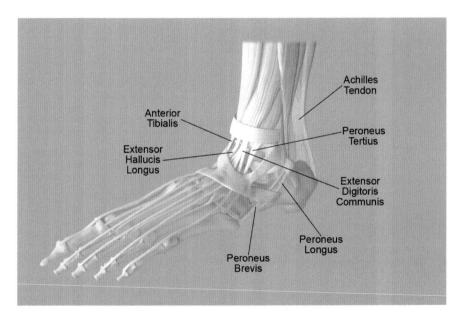

Fig. 4.3 Ankle Tendons.

4.2 Biomechanics

4.2.1 Kinematics

Ankle movement is a complex three dimensional motion, as illustrated in Fig. 4.4
[1], with infinity of instant axes of tibiotalar rotation, as is the case in all condylar
joints. Fortunately, for purposes of analysis and design the complex motion

degrees can be reasonably approximated by a planar plantar - dorsiflexion [2], axial (Internal - External) rotation and inversion-eversin.

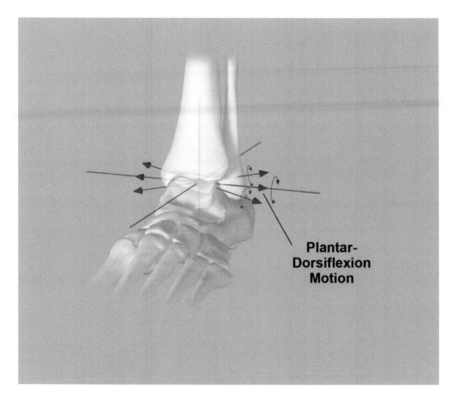

Fig. 4.4 Infinity of Instantaneous Axes of Tibiotalar Rotation [1].

The five degrees of freedom associated with the tibiotalar joint are:

Plantar - dorsiflexion; which is the principal motion of the joint.

Axial rotation; which; motion is limited primarily by the mortise and ligaments of the ankle.

Inversion - Eversion (I-E); which motion is limited by the ligaments and the tibiotalar articulating surfaces.

Anterior - posterior (A-P) translation; which motion is limited by the ligaments and the tibiotalar articulating surfaces.

Medial - Lateral (M-L) translation; which motion is limited by the mortise.

The first two are primarily associated with ankle motion and the remaining primarily with ankle stability.

These are illustrated in Fig. 4.5.

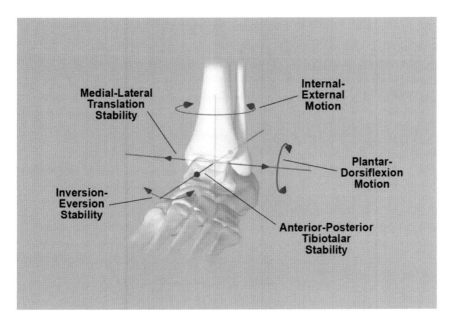

Fig. 4.5 Degrees of Movement and Stability.

4.2.1.1 Plantar - Dorsiflexion

The normal plantar - dorsiflexion range in level walking is typically about 25°-35°, as illustrated in Fig. 4.6.

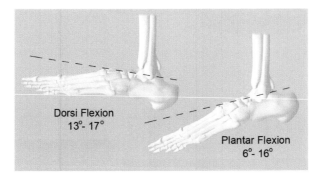

Fig. 4.6 Plantar and Dorsiflexion in the Normal Ankle During Walking.

If limited it adversely affects ankle function and can produce undesirable loading on the prosthesis, ligaments and bone fixation interface.

4.2.1.2 Axial Rotation

Normal axial rotation is about +5° to -3° during walking as shown in Fig. 4.7. Other activities can produce a maximum rotation of about 16° [3-5]. Any restriction of this motion is also undesirable as it produces undesirable torque on the prosthesis and bone fixation interface.

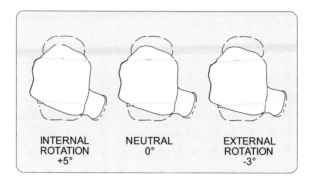

Fig. 4.7 Axial Rotation in the Normal Ankle During Walking.

4.2.2 Stability

The tibiotalar joint is stable and, thus, is constrained against significant anterior-posterior, medial-lateral and inversion - eversion motion. There are two types of stability: intrinsic stability provided by the shape of the articulating surfaces and extrinsic stability provided by soft tissues.

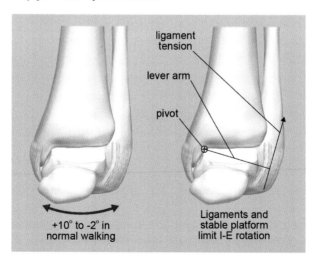

Fig. 4.8 Inversion-Eversion During Walking and stabilizing elements.

4.2.2.1 Inversion-Eversion

Normal inversion - eversion is about +10° to -2° during walking although most of this motion is in the subtalar joint [3-5]. Inversion - eversion stability is provided by the tibiotalar ligaments and the width of the tibiotalar articulating surface as shown in Fig. 4.8.

4.2.2.2 Anterior-Posterior

Anterior - posterior stability is primarily extrinsic and is provided by the ankle ligaments. Some intrinsic stability is also present as shown in Fig. 4.9.

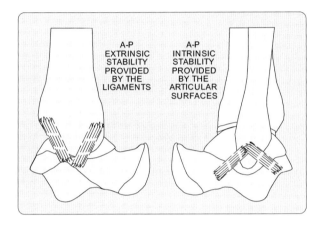

Fig. 4.9 A-P Stability of the Tibiotalar Joint.

4.2.2.3 Medial - Lateral

Medial - lateral stability is almost entirely intrinsic and is provided by the ankle mortise as shown in Fig. 4.10.

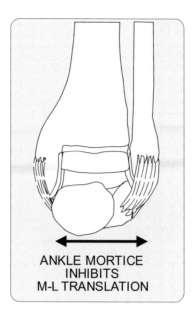

Fig. 4.10 M-L Stability of the Tibiotalar Joint.

There is, however, about 2mm of M-L motion in the normal ankle [3, 4].

4.2.3 Forces

Tibiotalar compressive forces have been estimated to exceed four times body weight during normal walking. The posterior shearing forces are estimated to be about 80% of body weight [3] as illustrated in Fig. 4.11.

The joint compression force is carried primarily by the tibiotalar articulating surfaces and partially by the talofibular joint. The A-P shearing force is carried by theses surfaces and the ligaments. The M-L shearing forces are carried by the malleolar articulation and I-E torques by the articulating surfaces and ligaments.

The combination of the axial compression and shearing forces produce a peak resultant force vector on the tibiotalar joint which is posteriorly inclined relative to the tibial axis as illustrated in Fig. 4.12.

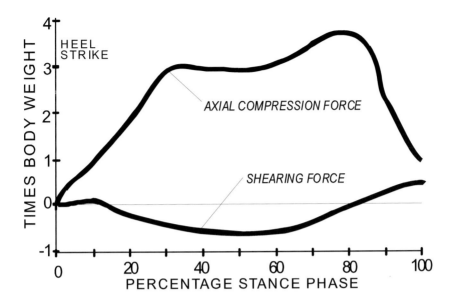

Fig. 4.11 Compressive Force in the Tibiotalar Joint [3].

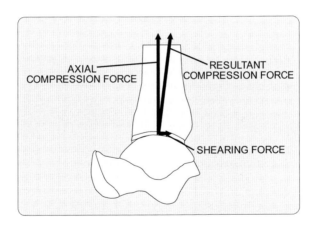

Fig. 4.12 Force Vectors in the Tibiotalar Joint.

4.3 Pathology

Disease processes involving the ankle joint are usually classified into congenital, metabolic, neuro-muscular, infectious, autoimmune and post-traumatic.

4.3.1 Congenital

Incomplete or poor embryonic development of the ankle can result from congenital anomalies such as "club foot" or "vertical talus". These disruptions in normal development can lead to multiple surgical corrections or amputation in severe cases to provide a limb capable of normal locomotion.

4.3.2 Metabolic

Bone disorders involving deficiencies in calcium metabolism secondary to hormonal, genetic or nutritional imbalance can affect the integrity of the bones and ligaments of the ankle, leading to joint destruction or mal alignment. Such disorders need to be accurately diagnosed and treated with appropriate medical management in addition to consideration of possible corrective foot and ankle surgery.

4.3.3 Neuromuscular

Diseases affecting the nerves and muscles of the leg and foot generally cause significant joint disturbances. Neural disorders such as Charcot-Marie Tooth disease (peroneal atrophy) can cause "high arch" of the foot which can complicate an on-going ankle condition. Neuromuscular disorders can severely affect the alignment of the foot and ankle and often require arthrodeses to control these deformities.

4.3.4 Infectious

Sepsis of the ankle from any gram positive or gram negative bacteria can result in destruction of the ankle joint, known as septic arthritis. These joints are at significant risk of re-infection and severe pain is usually managed by ankle fusion in neutral position. An ancient infection (greater than 20 years ago) in an otherwise healthy and immune competent patient may allow for joint replacement, but the risk of re-infection remains high.

4.3.5 Autoimmune

Arthritis of the ankle can be a result of autoimmune disorders such as rheumatoid or psoriatic arthritis which can completely destroy the articular cartilage. Evidence suggests that osteoarthritis has a genetic component that may be related to an autoimmune phenomenon as well. In any event, these arthritic conditions have a similar end-stage pathology, which makes them suitable candidates for joint replacement or fusion to improve their function.

4.3.6 Post-Traumatic

Fractures, dislocations or severe ligament injuries can compromise ankle joint function and in many cases cause severe cartilage destruction, similar to osteoarthritis. In patients with proper hind foot alignment and reconstructable ligaments, ankle joint replacement offers an improved alternative to ankle fusion. An x-ray of post-traumatic ankle arthritis is seen in Fig. 4.13.

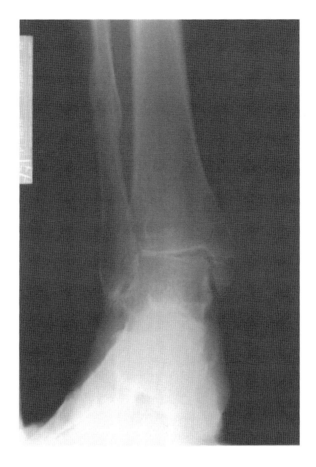

Fig. 4.13 Post-Traumatic Arthritis.

4.4   Total Ankle Replacement

4.4.1   Design Evolution

4.4.1.1   First Generation Designs

a) The Smith Ankle
This design was developed at Duke University in the early 1970's. It is a domed shaped unconstrained, ball and socket, cemented device with a stainless steel tibial component and an UHMWPe talar component [6].

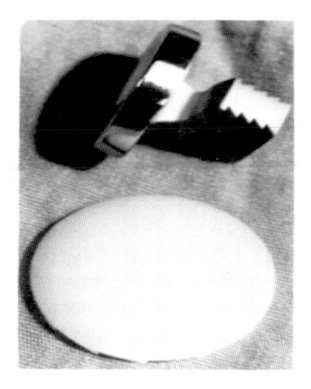

Fig. 4.14 Smith Total Ankle Replacement.

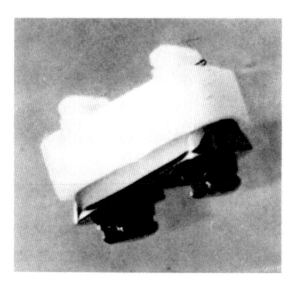

Fig. 4.15 Mayo Total Ankle Replacement.

b) The Mayo Clinic Ankle

This ankle was developed in 1974. It is a two part, fixed bearing, highly constrained, cemented design with a stainless steel talar and UHMWPe tibial component [7].

c) The NJ Fixed Bearing Ankle

The first ankle developed by the authors was a cylindrical design with congruent articulating surfaces [8]. It is a two piece device with a Co-Cr tibial component and an UHMWPe talar component. This design is shown in Fig. 4.16. It was first implanted in 1974.

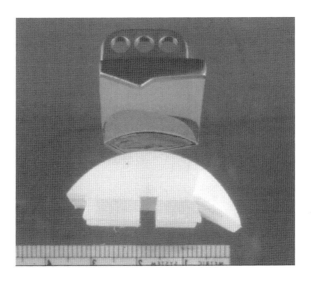

Fig. 4.16 NJ Cylindrical Ankle Replacement [8].

d) Others

Many other first generation designs were tried clinically. Ref. [9] discusses many of the first generation designs. Section 4.4.2.1 provides clinical information on the Oregon, Irvine, Beck-Steffee and TPR ankles.

4.4.1.2 Second Generation Designs

Problems with constrained Mayo Clinic [10-14] and NJ fixed bearing [15] design and the need to have congruent articulating contact lead to the adaption of the mobile bearing concept, first used by the authors in the shoulder in 1974 [16], to the ankle.

It has been found from extensive clinical experience with ankle replacement on the part of users of the Buechel-Pappas Ankle Replacement that almost all pathology encountered where replacement is indicated, is associated with the talar dome and its corresponding distal tibial articulating surface. The malleolar articulations are usually viable as are the ankle ligaments.

For such pathology it seems undesirable to remove any viable articulation and structure and desirable to retain them and their function. Furthermore, it is desirable to minimize bone loss associated with any procedure to implant a joint replacement. Thus, a resurfacing device that replaces essentially only the degenerated superior surface of the talar dome and its corresponding distal tibial articulating surface seems most appropriate.

Furthermore, to provide sufficient load bearing capacity, a congruent, mobile bearing is needed if the joint is to provide needed congruent articulation and yet avoid over constraint by providing needed motions such as axial rotation.

a) The B-P Trunion Total Ankle Replacement
The rotating trunion device of Fig. 4.17 was developed on these principles. It allowed axial rotation with congruity. This device was first implanted in 1976 in two patients and it worked well clinically.

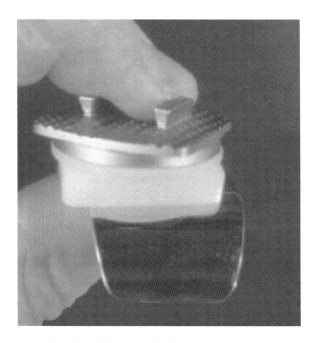

Fig. 4.17 B-P Trunion Total Ankle Replacement.

b) The LCS Meniscal Bearing Total Ankle Replacement
It became apparent that eliminating the intrinsic A-P constraint would provide a more accommodating, mobile joint without substantially compromising A-P stability. This lead to the development of the LCS or B-P Mark I Meniscal Bearing Ankle Replacement, an improved meniscal bearing device, shown in Fig. 4.18. It was first implanted in 1978 [17].

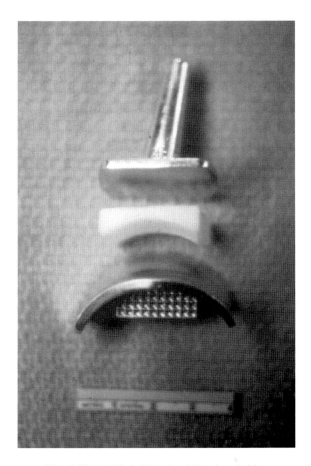

Fig. 4.18 B-P Mark I Meniscal Bearing Ankle.

This ankle is a three part design consisting of Cobalt-Chromium talar and tibial components with in interlaying bearing of UHMWPe. It was available in six sizes and intended for cemented fixation.

c) The S.T.A.R. Meniscal Bearing Total Ankle Replacement
This ankle is a three part design consisting of Cobalt-Chromium talar and tibial components with in interlaying bearing of UHMWPe. It resurfaces the gutters. Originally it was intended for use with cement, but in later forms it was biologically fixed without cement [18, 19]. It is the only mobile bearing ankle approved for sale in the United States of America. The meniscal bearing version was first implanted in 1986.

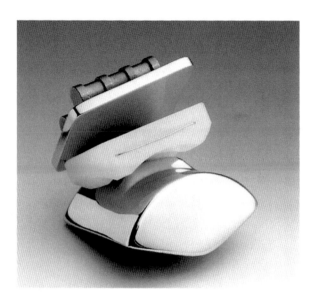

Fig. 4.19 S.T.A.R. Meniscal Bearing Total Ankle Replacement.

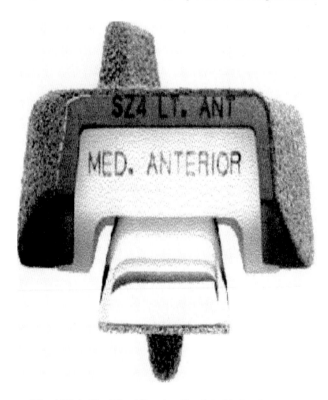

Fig. 4.20 Agility Fixed Bearing Total Ankle Replacement.

d) The Agility Fixed Bearing Total Ankle Replacement

Although the Agility [28] is considered by some a second generation design it is, in fact, more closely related to the first generation devices in performance and function. It is an advance over first generation devices primarily due to its use of biological fixation as opposed to the cemented fixation of the earlier designs. Although the device is clearly intended for biological fixation and is so used, it is curious that it is approved by the U.S. FDA only for cemented use.

This device is sold almost exclusively in the United States of America since the United States FDA made approval of mobile bearing devices quite difficult. It remained the only ankle replacement legally sold in the United States until the PMA approval of the S.T.A.R.in 2009. The Agility was first implanted in 1984 although it was not available commercially until 1994.

(e) Others

Many other designs such as the Hintegra, ACS, TOPAZ (INBONE), BOX, Salto and other all of which are mobile bearing designs except in versions modified for sale in the United States of America [21] have also been used clinically.

4.4.1.3 Third Generation Designs

a) The B-P Meniscal Total Ankle Replacement Mark II

This design is a major redesign of the LCS Total Ankle Replacement. It uses a much deeper sulcus and dual fin, rather than a central single fin talar fixation.

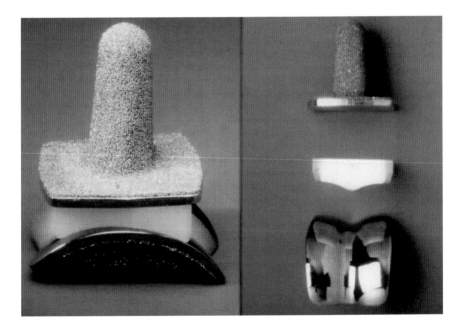

Fig. 4.21 B-P Meniscal Total Ankle Replacement Mark II.

This dual fin arrangement is employed to reduce the risk of talar subsidence. The AP dimension of the tibial plate is also significantly increased to provide greater bone coverage [22].

This is considered a third generation device since the device uses biological fixation and the metallic parts are titanium alloy coated with a propriety TiN coating. This coating overcomes the primary disadvantage of titanium alloy, its relatively poor abrasion resistance, by providing a surface and substrate superior to Co-Cr alloys in every important property.

b)   The B-P Meniscal Total Ankle Replacement Mark III

The Mark III differs from the Mark II in that it uses dual peg rather than dual fin fixation. The dual pegs are simpler to implant, but more importantly, they require less talar bone loss thus, reducing the risk of talar subsidence.

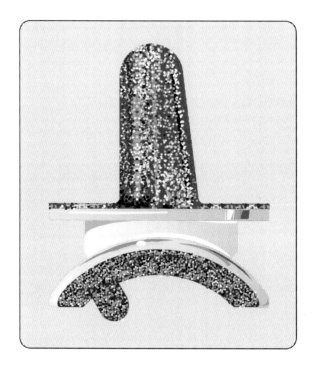

Fig. 4.22 B-P Mark III Total Ankle Replacement.

4.4.2   Evaluation

4.4.2.1   Clinical Outcomes of 1st Generation Total Ankle Arthroplasty

On Friday, July 2, 1982, in the Federal Register, Vol. 47, No. 128, the FDA published the proposed Rules for 888.3110; Docket No. 78N-3060; Ankle joint metal/polymer semi-constrained prosthesis [23]. The Orthopaedic Device Classification Panel's recommendations found that there was sufficient scientific evidence to support a Class II designation. (See section XI. Regulatory History: *Regulatory History of the ankle joint metal/polymer non-constrained prosthesis*). The Panel based its recommendation on four oral presentations based upon four semi-constrained ankles presented to the Panel. These presentations described and presented the relatively short-term clinical results of the following devices:

a) The Oregon ankle prosthesis presented by Dr. Harry Groth.
b) The Irvine ankle prosthesis presented by Dr. Theodore Waugh.
c) The Beck-Steffee ankle prosthesis presented by Dr. Arthur Steffee.
d) The TPR ankle prosthesis presented by Dr. Paul Thompson.

In the above studies the patient populations are different for each study.

The FDA agreed with the panel's recommendations and sought additional data and information on the safety and effectiveness of these devices. The FDA cited the following studies on two additional devices which are summarized below. For the Mayo ankle prosthesis:

Stauffer RN; Total joint arthroplasty. The ankle. *Mayo Clin Proc* 1979 Sep; 54(9): 570-5

The Mayo clinic developed a prosthetic ankle joint replacement. The Mayo total ankle replacement is a metal-on-polyethylene, congruent, constrained prosthesis. Analysis of 94 patients (102 ankle prostheses) revealed good clinical results in patients with rheumatoid arthritis and in older persons with posttraumatic degenerative disease. Younger, more active patients in the latter category had more disappointing results. Further design development is under way to improve range-of-motion characteristics, decrease constraint forces, and improve bone fixation of the prosthetic components [7].

For the Scholz ankle prosthesis:

Scholz KC: Total ankle arthroplasty using biological fixation components compared to ankle arthrodesis. *Orthopedics* 1987 Jan; 10(1):125-31.

When conservative measures fail to alleviate pain and disability of ankle joint disease, tibiotalar arthrodesis is the present accepted surgical treatment. Unfortunately, ankle arthrodesis also carries a significant rate of complications and the success rate does not parallel the results of hip and knee joint arthroplasties. A large percentage of ankle arthrodesis remain painful, and function is not normal. There is no satisfactory "salvage procedure" to a painful ankle fusion. Patients with primary ankle arthritis tend to develop bilateral ankle involvement as well as involvement of the subtalar and midtarsal joints; bilateral ankle fusion results in a severe handicap to gait and function. Total ankle arthroplasty using cement fixation remains controversial. Continued use of polymethylmethacrylate and additional design changes do not appear to be the answer to possible ankle joint replacement.

He concluded that the initial success using the PCA concept of biological cementless fixation of the Scholz total ankle prosthetic components appears to offer a new dimension in the success of total ankle arthroplasty [24].
The FDA also cited an additional reference on the Irvine ankle:

> Waugh TR; Evanski PM; McMaster WC; Irvine ankle arthroplasty. Prosthetic design and surgical technique. *Clin Orthop* 1976 Jan-Feb ;(114): 180-4.

> The Irvine total ankle arthroplasty is presented for highly selected cases. The design stems from investigations on the anatomical and biomechanical characteristics of the human ankle joint. The prostheses are inserted through an anterior approach. Full weight-bearing is well tolerated within a few days. The immediate results on 20 ankles are most encouraging [25].

It may be seen that the decisions of the panel and the FDA to designate semi-constrained ankles as class II were founded on relatively short-term encouraging results of early ankle designs based on presentations and publications of the developers of these ankles. Longer-term studies, however, clearly demonstrate that these ankle types are failures.

Consider the longer-term experience with the Mayo ankle prosthesis based on reports by several authors including Refs:

> Stauffer RN; Segal NM: Total ankle arthroplasty: four years' experience. *Clin Orthop* 1981 Oct ;(160): 217-21

> A review of 102 Mayo total ankle arthroplasties performed during a four-year period revealed that complications occurred in 41%. 22% with impingement of various types 6.9% with loosening and 2.9% with deep sepsis. The best results were obtained in patients with rheumatoid arthritis and those with posttraumatic osteoarthritis who were older than 60 years of age.

> They concluded that total ankle arthroplasty currently should not be considered in patients with posttraumatic osteoarthritis who are younger than 60 years old. Also, arthrodesis remains the only acceptable method of treatment in these individuals. Therefore, total ankle arthroplasty seems indicated in patients who have significant ankle joint disability secondary to rheumatoid arthritis and in elderly patients with disabling posttraumatic degeneration whose physical demands are limited [10].

> Lachiewicz PF; Inglis AE; Ranawat CS: Total ankle replacement in rheumatoid arthritis. *J Bone Joint Surg Am* 1984 Mar; 66(3): 340-3

> Fifteen single-axis arthroplasties were implanted in patients suffering from rheumatoid arthritis. Fourteen were of the Mayo type and one was of the Buchholz type. After an average follow-up of thirty-nine months seven ankles were rated excellent and eight, good. The relief of pain was gratifying in all of the patients, only four patients having residual slight pain with starting activity. The average gain in the range of motion was 9 degrees. No patient had loosening that required reoperation, although radiolucent lines

were seen in eleven ankles. Thirteen of the fifteen ankles had moderate to severe arthritic changes in the talonavicular, subtalar, or other intertarsal joints. They concluded that the early results were encouraging [11].

Kitaoka H.B. et al: Survivorship Analysis of the Mayo Total Ankle Arthroplasty. *The Journal of Bone and Joint Surgery* 76-A: 974-979, July 1994.

From 1974 until the end of 1988, 204 primary Mayo total ankle arthroplasties were performed at the Mayo Clinic. By means of actuarial analysis, the study determined that the cumulative rates of survival with failure (defined as removal of the implant) as the end point. The average duration of follow-up was nine years (range, two to seventeen years). By applying the Cox proportional-hazards general linear model, two independent variables were identified and associated with a significantly higher risk of failure. These variables were a previous operative procedure on the ipsilateral foot or ankle and an age of 57 years or less. The overall cumulative rate of survival at five, ten, and fifteen years was 79, 65, and 61 per cent, respectively. The probability of an implant being in situ at ten years was 42 per cent for patients who were 57 years old or less and who had had previous operative treatment of the ipsilateral ankle or foot and 73 per cent for those who were more than 57 years old and who had had no such previous operative treatment.

The study concluded that it is not recommended to use the Mayo total ankle arthroplasty, particularly in younger patients who have had a previous operative procedure on the ipsilateral ankle or foot [14].

Kitaoka HB; Patzer GL: Clinical results of the Mayo total ankle arthroplasty. *J Bone Joint Surg Am* 1996 Nov; 78(11): 1658-64.

Two hundred and four primary Mayo total ankle arthroplasties were performed in 179 patients at the Mayo Clinic from 1974 through 1988. The clinical result was evaluated after 160 arthroplasties in 143 patients who had been followed for two years or more (mean, nine years; range, two to seventeen years). The result was good for thirty-one ankles (19 per cent), fair for fifty-five (34 per cent), and poor for seventeen (11 per cent); fifty-seven arthroplasties (36 per cent) were considered to be a failure (defined as removal of the implant). Adequate preoperative and follow-up radiographs were available for 101 ankles (eighty-nine patients). There was radiographic evidence of loosening of eight tibial components (8 per cent) and fifty-eight talar components (57 per cent), but we found no association between the clinical and radiographic results. Complications occurred after nineteen (12 per cent) of the 160 arthroplasties, and ninety-four additional reoperations were necessary after sixty six (41 per cent) [12].

The study concluded that ankle arthroplasty is not recommended with a constrained Mayo implant for rheumatoid arthritis or osteoarthrosis of the ankle.

Unger AS; Inglis AE; Mow CS; Figgie HE: Total ankle arthroplasty in rheumatoid arthritis: a long-term follow-up study. *Foot Ankle* 1988 Feb; 8(4): 173-9

Twenty-one patients with rheumatoid arthritis were implanted with Mayo total ankle arthroplasties and had a minimum of 2 yr follow-up were reported. Of the original 21 patients, 17 were available for review. Twenty-three ankle replacements with an average follow-up of 5.6 yr were studied. On follow-up 2 ankles were rated excellent, 13 were rated good, 4 were rated fair, and 4 were rated poor. Thus, 83% were satisfactory on follow-up. Radiographic analysis revealed migration and settling of the talar component in 14 of 15 cases. Bone cement radiolucencies were found in 14 of 15 cases. Bone cement radiolucencies were found in 14 of 15 tibial components with tilting in 12 of these components. The postoperative position of the implant did not correlate with the development of radiolucencies or migration of the implant [13].

Thus, clearly the Mayo ankle prosthesis must be considered a failure.
  Next consider the Irvine device:

Evanski PH; Waugh TR: Management of arthritis of the ankle: An alternative of arthrodesis. *Clin Orthop* 1977 Jan-Feb ;(122): 110-5

Twenty-eight Irvine ankle arthroplasties were implanted and evaluated on a 100-point ankle analysis scale preoperatively and postoperatively. The average preoperative score was 35 and the average postoperative score was 74. Significant improvement occurred in function, pain relief and range of motion. The average follow-up period for these patients was 9 months. Complications included wound-healing problems in 3 patients. Mal-alignment of the prosthesis occurred in 2 other patients; one required revision. Ankle replacement failed in 2 patients. One patient required a fusion; the other an amputation following occlusion of the posterior tibial artery after surgery.

They concluded that at the present time, ankle replacement appears to be an acceptable alternative to ankle arthrodesis. Yet warned that the number in each group is small and that it does not appear that the procedure has merit for the treatment of ankle arthritis from such diverse causes as trauma, rheumatoid arthritis, aseptic necrosis of the talus and talectomy [26].

The Beck-Steffee device was similarly unsuccessful as demonstrated in:

Wynn A.H. et al: Long-term Follow-up of Conaxial (Beck-Stefee) Total Ankle Arthroplasty. *Foot and Ankle* 13: 303-306, Jul/Aug 1992.

Between 1975 and 1977, 30 patients with traumatic arthritis or rheumatoid arthritis underwent 36 Beck-Steffee Conaxial ankle replacements. Thirty-two were primary replacements and four were revisions of previous ankle arthroplasties. Twelve patients had traumatic osteoarthritis and 18 patients had rheumatoid arthritis. The average age at operation of patients with rheumatoid arthritis was 61 years (range 28-67 years) and with osteoarthritis was 52.9 years (range 32-72 years). The average follow-up was 10.8 years, with a range of 10 to 13 years. Early postoperative complications included wound dehiscence in 39% of patients (14 patients), deep wound infection in 6%, fractures of the medial or lateral malleolus in 22%, and painful talofibular impingement in 14%. At 2-year follow-up, 27% of the ankle replacements were loose. Sixty percent were loose at 5 years and 90% were loose at the 10-year follow-up. Ten patients had implant removal and attempted fusion. Six, or 60%, fused in an average of 5 months. Of those patients who achieved ankle fusion, four had internal fixation and iliac crest auto grafting, one had a Charnley compression apparatus with allograft bone, and one had internal fixation with allograft bone.

The study concluded that the constrained Conaxial ankle replacement should no longer be implanted because of a 90% loosening rate at 10 years and an overall complication rate of 60% [27].

The TPR ankle prosthesis is also unsuccessful as demonstrated by:

Jensen NC; Kroner K: Total ankle joint replacement: a clinical follow-up. *Orthopedics* 1992 Feb; 15(2): 236-9

The TPR total ankle joint replacement system (Smith & Nephew Richards) was implanted in 30 ankles in 25 patients. Twenty-three ankles in 18 patients were followed; 21 had rheumatoid arthritis and two had osteoarthritis. The average age at surgery was 62 years (range: 37 to 77), and the average follow up was 59 months (range: 37 to 89). The improvement was especially obvious with respect to pain and function. The average walking distance improved from 260 m preoperatively to 975 m postoperatively.

The study concluded that even though there was some improvement with respect to pain and function, the results of the study are disappointing in comparison to studies of ankle arthrodesis [28].

In addition several other semi-constrained ankle prostheses have been unsuccessful. These include the ICLH ankle device the clinical experience of which is reported by:

Herberts P; Goldie IF; Korner L; Larsson U; Lindborg G; Zachrisson BE: Endoprosthetic arthroplasty of the ankle joint: A clinical and radiological follow-up. *Acta Orthop* Scand 1982 Aug; 53(4): 687-96

Eighteen ICLH ankle arthroplasties were implanted in 16 patients. They were followed up after 15 to 52 months postoperatively (mean 36 months) by a review of the records, and clinical and radiological examinations. Five arthroplasties were performed for osteoarthrosis and 13 for rheumatoid arthritis. The overall clinical result was rated excellent in 2, good in 8, fair in 6, and poor in 2 joints. In osteoarthritic joints the results were somewhat poorer, no patient obtaining a rating of excellent but 2 of good, 2 of fair, and one of poor. Radiolucent zones greater than 2 millimeters were seen around the tibial component in 7 cases. Loosening defined as radiographic signs of movement between the prosthetic components and bone was present in 4 cases.

They concluded that the high occurrence of obvious loosening and large radiolucent zones indicates that mechanical problems will be encountered frequently in the future and that ankle arthroplasty has a definite place in the treatment of severe arthritis in rheumatoid patients [29].

Helm R; Stevens J: Long-term results of total ankle replacement. *J Arthroplasty* 1986; 1(4): 271-7

Nineteen ICLH total ankle replacements were implanted in 18 patients with rheumatoid or other inflammatory arthritis. After a mean follow-up period of 54.4 months (minimum, 24 months), three arthroplasties had failed, all because of loosening.

The study concluded that although all of the remaining patients were improved in terms of pain and function, there was radiographic evidence of loosening in a further eight patients [30].

Bolton-Maggs BG; Sudlow RA; Freeman MA: Total ankle arthroplasty: A long-term review of the London Hospital experience. *J Bone Joint Surg Br* 1985 Nov; 67(5): 785-90

Sixty-two ICLH total ankle arthroplasties were performed between 1972 and 1981. Forty-one of these have been reviewed clinically after an average follow-up of five and a half years; only 13 can be described as satisfactory. The complications encountered in all 62 arthroplasties are detailed, the most significant being superficial wound healing problems, talar collapse, and loosening of the components; 13 prosthetic joints have already been removed and arthrodesis attempted. The management of the complications is discussed.

The study concluded that in view of the high complication rate and the generally poor long-term clinical results, it is recommended that arthrodesis be the treatment of choice for the painful stiff arthritic ankle, regardless of the underlying pathological process [31].

And the Smith ankle and other semi-constrained devices reported by:

Dini AA; Bassett FH: Evaluation of the early result of Smith total ankle Replacement. *Clin Orthop* 1980 Jan-Feb; (146): 228-30

The Smith total ankle replacement was performed in 21 joints. During a 3-year period, the function was good in 50% of the patients with traumatic degenerative arthritis and 40% with rheumatoid arthritis.

The study concluded that improper technique; infection and component loosening were the most common causes of failure in 11 patients, with fair to poor prognosis [6].

Takakura Y; Tanaka Y; Sugimoto K; Tamai S; Masuhara K: Ankle arthroplasty: A comparative study of cemented metal and uncemented ceramic prostheses. *Clin Orthop* 1990 Mar ;(252): 209-16

From 1975 to 1980, Thirty Takakura cemented total ankle arthroplasties were implanted using metal/polyethylene prosthesis in twenty-eight patients with painful arthritis. However, because loosening and sinking of the prosthesis were significant, a ceramic total prosthesis was designed in 1980 to be used without cement. Between 1980 and 1987, 39 ankles in 35 patients with osteoarthritis, rheumatoid arthritis, and hemophilic arthritis were replaced using the ceramic prosthesis. Out of 39 ankles, nine were replaced with cement and 30 without cement. The follow-up period for the cemented metal and ceramic cases ranged from 13.4 to 6.2 years, with an average of 8.1 years, and for uncemented ceramic cases from 1.2 to 6.4 years, with an average of 4.1 years. Based on a rating scale for ankle evaluation, 27% of the cemented cases and 67% of the uncemented cases are satisfactory. Five metal ankles and one ceramic ankle were reoperated upon, with one revision and five arthrodeses performed.

The study concluded that ceramic total ankle arthroplasty, performed without cement, has to date provided mostly excellent stable results [32].

Kofoed H; Sorensen TS Ankle arthroplasty for rheumatoid arthritis and osteoarthritis: prospective long-term study of cemented replacements. *J Bone Joint Surg Br* 1998 Mar; 80(2):328-32

Fifty-two cemented ankle arthroplasties were implanted for painful osteoarthritis (OA) (25) or rheumatoid arthritis (RA) (27) using an ankle prosthesis with a near-anatomical design. The patients were assessed radiologically and clinically for up to 14 years using an ankle scoring system. The preoperative median scores were 29 for the OA group and 25 for the RA group and at ten years were 93.5 and 83, respectively. Six ankles in the OA group and five in the RA group required revision or arthrodesis. Survivorship analysis of the two groups showed no significant differences with 72.7% survival for the OA group and 75.5% for the RA group at 14 years [33].

Kofoed H Cylindrical cemented ankle arthroplasty: a prospective series with long-term follow-up. *Foot Ankle Int* 1995 Aug; 16(8):474-9

From 1981 to 1985, twenty-eight ankle arthroplasties were implanted using a congruent and cylindrical ankle design. The talus component was an anatomically shaped cap to cover the talus dome and the facets. The tibial component was congruent toward the talus and had two parallel bars on the back for fixation into the distal tibia. The diagnosis was osteoarthritis in 15 cases and rheumatoid arthritis in 11 cases (two bilateral cases).

There occurred seven failures, giving a cumulative estimated survival rate of 70% for the prosthesis at 12 years [18].

Neufeld S.K. and Lee T. H.: Total Ankle Arthroplasty: Indications, Results, and Biomechanical Rationale. *American Journal of Orthopedics* 593-602, Aug 2000.

Many physicians today, are reluctant to opt for a total ankle replacement and advocate ankle arthrodesis. They conclude that an ankle replacement has generally poor long-term results and a high rate of complications.

This caution is warranted states Neufeld, when applied to early ankle replacement designs, "Published studies of early series with greater follow-up show that ankle arthroplasties did not provide lasting pain relief or improve function, and ultimately failed" [34].

These studies are summarized in the following Tables 4.1 and 4.2. The early optimism soon indicated in Table 4.1 gave way to failure as shown in Table 4.2:

Table 4.1 Short Term Follow-up: Cemented First Generation Total Ankle Arthroplasty.

Authors	Device*	Number of Cases	Diagnosis	Average Follow-up	Survival Rate (%)
Stauffer & Segal [10]	Mayo	102	SA (56), RA (43), OA (3)	1.9 yr	93
Lachiewlcz et al [11]	Mayo	15	RA (15)	3 yr	100
Herberts et al [29]	ICLH	21	RA (14), OA (7)	3 yr	86
Newton [35]	Newton	50	RA (10), OA (34), SA (6)	3 yr	(60), (38), (0)
Dini & Bassett [6]	Smith	5	RA (5)	2.5 yr	80
			SA (16)	2.1 yr	75
Evanski & Waugh [26]	Irvine	16	RA (5), OA (23)	9 mths	93

4.4.2.2   Analysis of the First Generation Total Ankle Designs

Although early ankle replacement designs were failures, this fact did not discourage designers. Development of newer designs continued since ankle arthrodesis is not a perfect solution to the problem of treating ankle arthritis. Arthrodesis can be fraught with complications such as non-union and mal-union and even in perfect alignment it has been proven to put increased stress on the knee, subtalar and midfoot regions [34].

Furthermore, Neufeld and Lee [34] state "the diminished overall motion and increased stresses on the remaining joints may lead to a poor result in an ankle arthrodesis. After a pan-talar arthrodesis, dorsiflexion is diminished by approximately 63% and plantar flexion by about 82%…an ankle fusion is helpful only initially and that eventual failure due to the subtalar or talocalcaneal joints becoming overstressed is inevitable. Therefore, a reliable ankle replacement system would be a welcome addition to orthopedic practice". The early ankle designs did not provide this due to their poor performance.

Table 4.2 Longer Term Follow-up: Cemented First Generation Total Ankle Arthroplasty.

Authors	Device*	Number of Cases	Diagnosis	Average Follow-up	Survival Rate (%)
Jensen and Kroner [28]	TPR	148	RA (21), OA (2), RA (125)	4.9 yr	48
Kitaoka et al [14]	Mayo	79	SA (65), OA (14)	5 yr, 10 yr, 15 yr	79, 65, 61
Kitaoka & Patzer [12]	Mayo	168	RA (96), SA (64), OA (8)	9 yr	64
Wynn & Wilde [27]	Beck-Steffee	30	RA (18), SA (12)	2 yr, 5 yr, 10 yr	73, 40, 10
Helm and Stevens [30]	ICLH	19	RA (19)	4.5 yr	83
Bolton-Maggs et al [31]	ICLH	62	RA (34), OA (13), SA (15)	5.5 yr	47
Unger et al [13]	Mayo	23	RA (23)	5.6 yr	65
Takakura et al [32]	Takakura Cemented	33	OA (20), RA (11), SA (2)	8.8 yr (metal), 6.7 yr (ceramic)	15
Kofoed & Sorensen [41]	2 piece (early) 3-piece (later)	52	OA (25), RA (27)	14 yr	75.5 (RA) 72.7 (OA)
Kofoed [18]	Cylindrical 2-piece Cemented	28	RA (13) OA (15)	12 yr	70

In addition Neufeld and Lee add "After early successes, the longer-term results bred failure". Lachiewicz et al [11] reported in 15 patients, with one of the most widely used prostheses, the Mayo ankle, with an average follow-up of 3.3 years and excellent results. When Unger and coworkers [13] reported in the same 15 patients with a longer follow-up of 6.2 years, deterioration in their clinical scores and radiographs was apparent.

Neufeld and Lee also state "Several reasons for the long-term failure of the early prostheses have been suggested. First, many original designs required excessive bone resections and relied on cement fixation onto soft cancellous bone. Constrained prostheses placed excessive stress on the cement-cancellous bone interface. Subsequently the main reason for their failure was aseptic loosening. Unconstrained prostheses…failure occurred due to malleolar and soft-tissue impingement…Therefore, the failure of early designs may have been caused by the lack of respect for the anatomy, kinematics, alignment and stability of the ankle joint".

Furthermore they state "They (early constrained designs) have failed to incorporate the biomechanical characteristics of the ankle joint…The design of the implant should permit effective transfer of joint loads, be inherently stable, allow ease of surgical implantation/removal with minimum bone loss, and have resistance to wear, creep, fatigue failure and compressive shear loading".

Therefore, despite encouraging early results, long-term studies proved that constrained ankle devices were not viable and were subsequently abandoned by the orthopaedic community in favor of arthrodesis. Yet, under the present FDA classification system they can still be manufactured and sold today. It may be true that, given the preliminary evidence of these early studies, that the Orthopedic Device Classification Panel in July 1982 were reasonable in classifying these devices as Class II, yet based on the long-term studies this is clearly no longer the case today. The FDA, however, still persist in employing this discredited classification.

4.4.2.3   Clinical Outcomes of Second Generation Total Ankle Arthroplasty

a) B-P Mark I (LCS) Total Ankle System (Shallow Sulcus)
The B-P Mark I ankle first implanted in 1978 was more successful than the typical semi-constrained devices. Unfortunately it suffered from a problem, which although unrelated to constraint, caused the device to be abandoned and redesigned. Below are summarized six mobile bearing clinical studies associated with this early mobile bearing design. These studies represent Mark I clinical performance over a twenty-year time span. The four studies are summarized as follows:

> Buechel FF, Buechel FF Jr., and Pappas MJ: Twenty Year Evaluation of Cementless Mobile-Bearing Total Ankle Replacements. *Clinical Orthop.* 424:19-26, 2004.

> There were 38 patients implanted with 40 Mark I (shallow sulcus) ankles over an eighteen-year time span. Mean age was 55 years. Using a strict ankle scoring system, twenty-eight (70%) patients reported good/excellent results. One patient developed a fracture of the loading plate. Two patients had tibial components revised as a result of excessive wear. No tibial components were noted as clinically loose, all revised tibial components were stable at time of revision. Bearing subluxation problems occurred in 10% of cases. Talar subsidence occurred in 15% of cases. Both were rectified by a revised design (see 5. The prototype: B-P TAR, deep sulcus). Cumulative survivorship using an endpoint of revision of any component was 74.2% at eighteen years.

> The author concluded that the mobile bearing greatly improved the ability of surgeons to replace ankles while minimizing wear and loosening problems. Design improvements, such as the deepening the sulcus while maintaining bispherical congruity of the bearing surface, have enhanced the longevity of the device [22].

> Buechel FF and Pappas MJ et al.: New Jersey Low-Contact Stress Ankle Replacement: Biochemical Rationale and Review of 23 Cementless Cases: Foot and Ankle, *American Orthopedic Foot and Ankle Society,* Vol. 8, No. 8, 1988, 279-290.

There were 21 patients implanted with 23 ankles. The mean age was 56 years. The follow-up period ranged from 24 months to 64 months with a mean of 35.3 months. The pre-operative ROM arc was 15 to 24 degrees. Post-operatively mean arc was 25 to 34 degrees. Postoperatively, 87% of ankles had no pain or, at most, mild pain and all had an improvement on their preoperative condition.

The author concluded unconstrained congruent bearing elements of the trochlear design appear to work well in patients throughout the 5-year period [17].

Keblish PA: Cementless Meniscal Bearing (Shallow Sulcus) TAR: *Multicenter Clinical Trial of 237. Unpublished.*

There were 237 patients implanted in 72 months. The mean age was 57 years. Survivorship was 90.7% and good to excellent results of 81.5% and 77% of patients had no/slight pain. 25 ankles were removed and 14 required arthrodesis.

The author concluded, "in order for total ankle replacement to gain general acceptance as a viable surgical option, several criteria must be met:

❖ Prosthetic design must permit optimal contact stress at the articulating surfaces and optimal fixation (preferably biological);
❖ Stability must be enhanced without compromising mobility;
❖ Strict criteria for surgical indications must be established;
❖ Arthrodesis must be a reasonable option as a salvage procedure (e.g. minimal bone resection)."

Cementless, meniscal bearing ankle systems fit these criteria [36].

Furthermore, "The complication rate is high…increased sensitivity in patient selection and surgical technique should decrease the complications and failure rate".

Doets HC: 6 (2-13) Year Results with the LCS/Buechel-Pappas Mobile Bearing Prosthesis. ERASS, 2002.

There were 58 prostheses implanted in 50 patients. Of these 20 were shallow-sulcus, the remaining number with the Buechel-Pappas prosthesis, 42 were women (8 bilateral) and 8 were men, 54 were diagnosed with rheumatoid arthritis, 3 with juvenile chronic arthritis and 1 with psoriatic arthritis. Mean age was 55 (22-77). Six patients (seven ankles) died of causes unrelated to the device. Ten had to be converted to arthrodesis, six for a varus or a valgus deformity and 3 for aseptic loosening of the tibial component and one for an early deep infection. Mean post-operative score improved from 37 to 74/100.

The author concluded that for polyarthritis the LCS/Buechel-Pappas TAP give good clinical results if correct alignment is achieved in surgery [37].

Doets HC: The Low Contact Stress/Buechel-Pappas Total Ankle Prosthesis: *Chapter 6 Current Status of Ankle Arthroplasty, Berlin, Springer 1998, Kofoed H., ed.*

There were 30 prostheses implanted in 28 patients, 20 shallow-sulcus, and the remaining number with the Buechel-Pappas prosthesis. The average age was 56 years. 25 of the number were diagnosed with rheumatoid arthritis the rest with juvenile chronic arthritis, psoriatic arthritis and osteoarthrosis. Three patients (four ankles) died of causes unrelated to the device. Four failed and were successfully converted to arthrodesis. Average post-operative score was 84/100.

The author concluded "Compared with two-component designs, the mobile bearing LCS/Buechel-Pappas TAP provides much better results, with low incidence of mechanical loosening." Furthermore, "With the STAR, also a three-component resurfacing design...similar good results have been reported. This demonstrates that in the ankle joint there is only place for a TAP, which uses a mobile bearing, and that the use of the two-component design is no longer indicated" [38].

San Giovanni T. et al: Long-term follow-up with second generation, cementless Total Ankle Replacement. *Annual meeting of the American Orthopedic Foot and Ankle Society (AOFAS), Summer 1999.*

There were 21 prostheses implanted in 16 patients. Mean follow-up 5.5 years. 18/21 had excellent results with no to mild pain. 3/21 had radiographic changes in component position. Two patients suffered talar subsidence and one a tibial component loosening. No polyethylene subluxation was noted. Three prostheses were considered failures. One prosthesis was removed secondary to deep infection (prosthesis revised). One had a polyethylene exchange for painful talar subsidence. A third prosthesis displayed tibial component loosening and will require revision or arthrodesis. The authors concluded: "The present study with intermediate-term follow-up demonstrates encouraging results with the use of a cementless, minimally constrained total ankle replacement...The overall patient satisfaction was high." [39].

As can be seen from the table below, putting aside the problems of talar subsidence and bearing subluxation there are few device related complications. The dominant complications are medical and surgical which can be dealt with by improvement in instrumentation and surgical techniques.

The four studies are summarized in Table 4.3 as follows:

Table 4.3 Clinical Data B-P Mark I (NJ LCS) Total Ankle Replacements.

	Buechel (22)	Buechel (17)	Keblish (36)	Doets (37)	Doets (38)	San Giovanni (39)
Number of cases	40 (38 Patients)	23	237	58	30 (28 patients)	21
M/F	Male = 20 Female = 20	Male = 12 Female = 11			Male = 2 Female = 26	
Age (mean)	55	56	57	55	56	-
Diagnosis	PTA= 21 (52.5%) OA= 7 (17.5%) RA= 9 (22%) Fusion= 3 (7.5%)	PTA= 10 (43.5%) OA= 4 (17.4%) RA= 6 (26.1%) AVN= 2(8.7%) Fusion= 1(4.3%)	PTA, OA, RA	RA, JCA, PA	RA= 25 (88%) JCA= 1 (4%) PA= 1 (4%) OA= 1 (4%)	RA
Follow-up	Mean 10 Yrs (2 –20 Yrs)	Mean 35 mths (24 - 64 mths)	Mean 45 mths (18 – 72 mths)	Avg. 6 Yrs (2 – 13 Yrs)	Avg. 6 Yrs (3 – 9 Yrs)	Mean 5.5 yrs (3.3-9.0 yrs)
Delayed Wound Healing	9 (23%)	4 (19%)	2 (1%)	0 (0%)	3 (10%)	-
Talar Subsidence	6 (15%)	0 (0%)	3 (2%)	0 (0%)	0 (0%)	2 (10%)
Bearing subluxation	4 (10%)	1 (5%)	11(5%)	0 (0%)	3 (10%)	0 (0%)
Severe bearing wear	4 (10%)	0 (0%)	17 (7%)	2 (3%)	0 (0%)	1 (5%)
Malleolar fracture	3 (8%)	1 (5%)	6 (11%)	-	5 (17%)	-
Infection	2 (5%)	1 (5%)	9 (4%)	1 (2%)	1 (3%)	2 (10%)
Reflex sympathic Dystrophy	2 (5%)	2 (10%)	1 (1%)	0 (0%)	0 (0%)	-
Varus/ Valgus Deformity	-	-	-	6 (10%)	-	-
Tibial loosening	0 (0%)	0 (0%)	6 (3%)	3 (5%)	1 (3%)	1 (5%)
Survivorship (Percentage)	74.2 (Kaplan-Meier) Revision for any reason at 20 yrs	100 (Kaplan-Meier) Revision for any reason at 5 yrs	90.7 (Kaplan-Meier) Revision for any reason	-	-	-
Average Overall Clinical Score (Percentage)	70 (NJOHAEF)	83.7 (NJOHAEF)	81.5 (NJOHAEF)	74 (NJOHAEF)	84 (NJOHAEF)	87 (AOFAS)

c)   The S.T.A.R. Total Ankle System

Clinical experience with what the FDA considers "non-constrained" devices are however favorable. Consider the studies of the S.T.A.R. device. These studies present the clinical result of the S.T.A.R. prosthesis over a ten-year time span. Four studies are as follows:

Valderrabano V, Hintermann B & Dick W: Scandinavian Total Ankle Replacement. *Clinical Orthop* 424:47-56, 2004

65 patients representing 68 S.T.A.R. arthroplasties were reviewed for 2-6 years. No infection occurred, no patients died during the follow-up. Early experience with the S.T.A.R. is encouraging, although more complications have been encountered than previously reported [40].

Schernberg F: Current results of Ankle Arthroplasty – European Multi-center Study of Cementless Ankle Arthroplasty. *Chapter 9, Current Status of Ankle Arthroplasty, Berlin, Springer 1998, Kofoed H., ed.*

131 STAR ankles were implanted in a multi-center study covering six European sites. There were eight failures after 1-year and 5 failures after 2 years. No failures were seen after the 2-year follow-up mark. The good results depended upon good patient selection and good technical management of the procedure [41].

Kofoed H: Scandinavian Total Ankle Replacement (STAR). *Clinical Orthop* 424:73-79, 2004.

58 patients with either rheumatoid arthritis or osteoarthritis were implanted with the STAR meniscal bearing ankle. Cement was used for 33 patients and Cementless for 25 and the mean follow up was 9.4 years. In the cemented group 9 patients failed and were revised or fused. In the cementless group 1 patient had revision surgery. Survivorship based on life tables showed a 70% survival rate at 12 years and 95.4% for the cementless group. Average clinical scores at the latest follow up were 74.2 ± 19.3 and 91.9 ± 7.4 respectively.

The authors concluded that 'unconstrained meniscal-bearing ankle prostheses should be uncemented' [42].

Kofoed H: Ankle Arthroplasty: Indications, Alignment, Stability and Gain in Mobility: Chapter 4, *Current Status of Ankle Arthroplasty,* Berlin, Springer 1998, Kofoed H., ed.

76 STAR devices were implanted. 44 had osteoarthrosis, 22 had rheumatoid arthritis, 4 talar necrosis, 4 psoriatic arthritis, and a conversion of a previous fusion. Five failed of the OA, RA diagnoses and all four of the AVN sufferers. Yet, despite the failures the current results are competitive with the best results of arthrodesis, without contracting secondary sub-talar problems.

The author concluded that for good and lasting results, alignment and stability are mandatory. The early designs were too constrained to give stability resulting in a transfer all stresses to the bone-cement interface, leading to excessive loosening. Also, the spheroid design led to reliance on ligaments without certainty of maintaining the ankle axis. Conversely, the 3-part design offers both alignment and stability without over constraint. They preserve both the axis of the ankle cylindrical motion and remain as anatomical as possible [43].

The four studies are summarized in Table 4.4 as follows:

Table 4.4 Clinical Data S.T.A.R. Total Ankle Replacement

Study	Valderrabano (40)	Schernburg (41)	Kofoed (42)	Kofoed (43)
Device	S.T.A.R. Mobile Bearing TAR	S.T.A.R. Mobile Bearing TAR	S.T.A.R. Mobile Bearing TAR	S.T.A.R. Mobile Bearing TAR
Number of cases	68 (65 Patients)	131	Cemented =33 Cementless = 25 Total 58	76
M/F	Male = 31 (48%) Female =34 (52%)		Male Cemented = 14 Female Cemented = 19 Male Cementless = 16 Female Cementless= 9	Male = 35 (46%) Female =41(54%)
Age (mean)	56	-	Cemented = 60 Cementless = 58	56
Diagnosis	PTA=48 (71%) RA = 11(16%) OA = 9 (13%)	OA, RA	Cemented RA = 13 Cemented OA = 20 Cementless RA = 3 Cementless OA = 22	OA = 44 (58%) RA = 22(29%) PA = 4 (6%) AVN = 4 (6%) Failed Fusion = 1(1%)
Follow-up	Mean 3.7 Year (2.4-6.2 years)	6 yrs	Cemented = 9.3 ± 2.7 Cementless = 9.5 ± 1.7	10 yrs
Delayed Wound Healing	-	-	-	-
Talar Subsidence	1 (4%)	-	-	-
Bearing subluxation	1 (4%)	-	-	-
Severe bearing wear	3 (13%)	-	Cementless 1(2%)	-
Malleolar fracture	0 (0%)	-	-	-
Infection	0 (0%)	-	-	-
Reflex sympathic Dystrophy	1 (6%)	-	Cemented 1(2%)	-
Tibial component loosening	2 (9%)	-	Cemented 6(10%) Cementless 1(2%)	-
Survivorship (%)	87 (After component related revision) at 6 yrs	87.3 (Kofoed, 1986) At 6 yrs	70 Cemented 95 Cementless (Revision/Removal for any reason) at 9 yrs	86.7 (Kofoed, 1986) (Revision for any reason) at 10 yrs
Average Clinical Score Overall (Percentage)	85 (AOFAS)	85 (Kofoed, 1986)	Cemented = 74.2 ± 19.3 Cementless = 91.9 ± 7.4	-

d) The Agility Total Ankle System
The following articles are examples of the high rate of complications associated with a semi-constrained device that is cleared by the FDA and legally marketed throughout the United States.

Saltzman CL et al: Surgeon Training and Complications in Total Ankle Arthroplasty. *Foot and Ankle Int.* Vol. 24, No. 6, pp.514-518, June 2003.

There were 26 patients in the study. The study assessed the problems with the initial use of ankle arthroplasty. 3 Groups were observed; Group 1 assessed 3 surgeons who were trained observing the surgeon/inventor; Group 2 assessed 3 surgeons who completed a structured, hands-on surgical training; Group 3 assessed 3 surgeons who were trained during a 1-year foot and ankle fellowship. The combined 3 groups reported 28 Syndesmosis non-unions, 19 Intraoperative complications, 7 Major revisions, 8 Syndesmosis Re-arthrodeses and 14 other secondary operations. Three Patients received a below the knee amputation.

The authors admitted that due to the small sample size the study had clear limitations. However, a relatively high complication rate could be the result of a 'high learning curve' [44].

Rippstein PF: Clinical experiences with three different designs of ankle prostheses. *Foot Ankle Clin N Am.* 7:817-931, 2002.

A total of 27 ankles were implanted in 25 patients. 19 PTA and 8 RA. Mean age 56.9 years. Mean follow-up 14.7 months. Eight revisions. Four seriously migrated. Two removed and ankle fused, one had tibial replacement, another was asymptomatic and left implanted. One early deep infection successfully treated. One case of complicated and painful tibial nerve neuropathy. Three revisions due to bony proliferation on the resected talus area, which was painfully impinging on the tibial component during dorsal extension. One Dwyer osteotomy performed as a result of medial ankle pain due to a varus malposition in the previously fused subtalar joint.

The author admitted that the high complication rate could be improved with further surgical experience, yet expressed serious concerns about the difficulty of performing any future potential fusion [45].

Pyevich, MT et al: Total ankle arthroplasty: A unique design. J. Bone Joint Surg. 80: 1410-1420, 1998.

There were 100 ankles were implanted in 95 patients. 12 patients died leaving 86 ankles. The average age was 63 years. Average follow-up 4.8 years. Five revisions. Twenty-one (24%) components had migrated. Twenty-eight ankles suffered delayed union of syndesmosis fusion and nine non-unions associated with the development of lysis around the tibial component. Non-union of the syndesmosis was also associated with the migration of the tibial component. One removal resulted in ankle fusion. 55% of ankles were not painful. 28% mildly painful. 93% were satisfactory to the patients.

The author concluded that early clinical results with the Agility were encouraging, although radiographic findings remained a cause for concern. Long-term studies will clarify as to whether delayed union or non-union of the syndesmosis is associated with an increased rate of clinically significant problems [46].

Spirt AA et al: Complications and Failure after Total Ankle Replacement. *J Bone Joint Surg Am.* 86-A(6):1172-1178, June 2004.

306 ankles were implanted in 303 patients. 85 patients (28%) underwent 127 reoperations for debridement of heterotopic bone (58), correction of axial malalignment (40),and component replacement (31). Survivorship with failure as an endpoint was 80%. Survivorship with reoperation as the endpoint was 54%.

The authors concluded that there was a relatively high rate of reoperation due to complications. Younger age was found to be a negative effect on reoperation and failure [47].

The four studies are summarized in Table 4.5. Of these studies, Spirit et al [47] is the most important since it is done by an independent group and has the largest number of cases. From these studies the Agility seems unacceptable for use in ankle replacement in the hands of many surgeons.

Somewhat better results are reported in a study of somewhat older patients of the developer of the Agility device (a mean 63 years of age vs. 53 in Spirt et al) by compensated evaluators not involved in patient treatment [48]. This study reports a survival rate (revision or arthrodesis as an end point) of about 95% at 5 years, about 88% at 9 years and about 63% at 12 years. A slightly earlier evaluation, in Ref. [42], of the results of these same patients shows a survival rate (revision as an endpoint) of about 90% at 5 years, 80% at 9 years and 61% at 12 years.

Table 4.5 Clinical Data on the Agility Total Ankle Replacement

Study	Saltzman (44)	Rippstein (45)	Pyevich (46)	Spirt (47)
Number of cases	90	27	85 (82 patients)	306
M/F	-	-	Male = 43 (52%) Female =39(48%)	Male = 52% Female = 49%
Age (mean)	GP 1 = 63 GP 2 = 56 GP 3 = 59	57	63	53
Diagnoses	OA= 73 (81%) RA =17 (19%)	PTA= 19 (70%) RA =8 (30%)	PTA= 44 (53%) OA= 19 (22%) RA =19 (22%) SA= 2 (2%) PA= 1 (1%)	PTA= 198 (65%) OA= 77(25%) Fusion Takedown =17(5.6%) RA =13 (4.2%) PTA/RA =1 (0.3%)
Follow-up	6 mths – 1 year	Mean 15 mths (5-22 mths)	Avg. 4.8 years (3-12 years)	Avg. 2.5 Years (2-6 years)
Delayed union of syndesmosis	Gp 1 = 10/26 (38%) Gp 2 = 13/26 (50%) gp 3 = 5/30 (17%)	-	28 (29%)	14(5%)
Revision fusion of syndesmosis	Gp 1 = 2/26 (8%) Gp 2 = 3/26 (10%) gp 3 = 3/26 (12%)	-	9 (9%)	14(5%)
Wound Dehiscence/ Debridement	Gp 1 = 6/30 (20%) Gp 2 = 3/30 (10%) GP 3 = 4/30(13%)	-	2 (2%)	69(23%)
Achilles tendon lengthening	Gp 1 = 2/30 (7%)	-	-	-
Component exchange/ removal	Gp 1 = 3/30 (10%) Gp 2 = 4/30 (13%)	4 (15%)	9 (9%)	31(10%)
Below Knee Amputation	Gp 1 = 1/30 (3%) Gp 2 = 2/30 (7%)	-	-	8(3%)
Malleolar fracture	Gp 1 = 6/30 (20%) Gp 2 = 3/30 (10%)	-	-	-
Infection	Gp 1 = 3/30 (10%) Gp 2 = 1/30 (3%)	1 (4%)	0 (0%)	11(4%)
Survivorship (%)	68 (using revision for any reason as an endpoint) at 1yr	-	-	80 (revision, arthrodesis or amputation as end point) at 6 yrs

4.4.2.4   Analysis of the Second Generation Total Ankle Designs

a) S.T.A.R.
Of the second generation designs the S.T.A.R. has the best clinical performance. Further, this device provides essentially normal gait [42]. This good performance is further evidenced by the approval of the PMA, based on a well controlled clinical trial, by the FDA allowing, for the first time, the sale of a mobile bearing ankle in the United Stated of America.

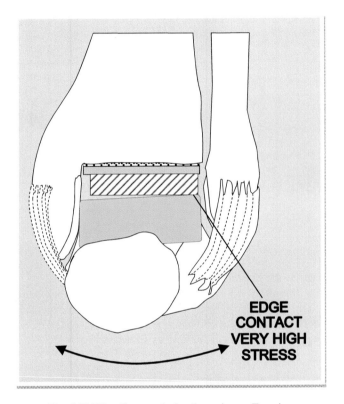

Fig. 4.23 Edge Contact during Inversion or Eversion.

However, the primary fault of the S.T.A.R. is that it loses congruity in the event of inversion or eversion as illustrated in Fig. 4.23.

b) The B-P Mark I (LCS)
The LCS design, although performing well in the short term, experienced degradation in performance with time. The most frequent cause of failure is related to talar subsidence.
This subsidence was due to several causes. The long fin allowed distal fixation to occur leading the stress protection of the proximal talus. This contributed to

atrophy and collapse of the talus leading to talar component subsidence and bearing extrusion and wear.

In examining the blood supply to the talus [50] it was concluded that the relatively long central fin may be disrupting blood supply excessively further contributing to talar necrosis and collapse. This failure mode is illustrated in Fig. 4.24.

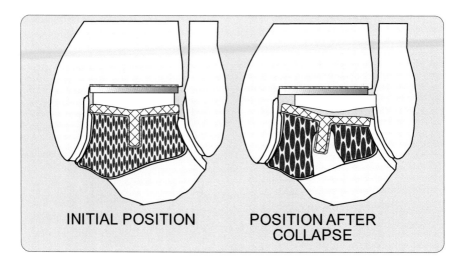

INITIAL POSITION   POSITION AFTER
                          COLLAPSE

Fig. 4.24 Failure Mode of the Mark I.

c) Agility Total Ankle Replacement

The Agility as originally commercially distributed by DePuy had four major design faults. The most important is that the contact stresses expected in the joint were in excess of the maximum allowable for the material [51, 52]. Secondly, the device did not provide normal I-E stability as shown in Fig. 4.25.

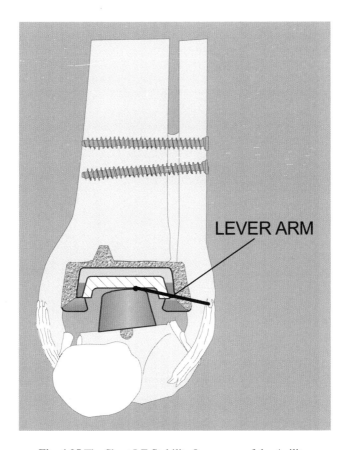

Fig. 4.25 The Short I-E Stability Lever arm of the Agility.

Thirdly, the talar component fails to cover much of the resected talar surface as illustrated in Fig. 4.26.

This lack of coverage substantially increases the stresses at the bone–prosthesis interface increasing the risk of loosening.

Finally, the Agility shifts the load normally carried by the talofibular joint to the tibiotalar joint, increasing loading on this joint, thereby, increasing wear and risk of loosening of the device.

Considering the nature of these design flaws the poor performance observed clinically is to be expected.

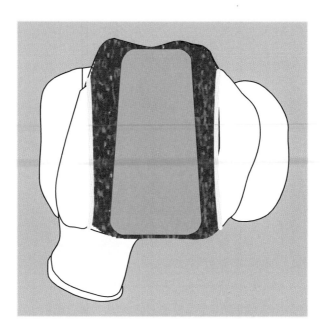

Fig. 4.26 Incomplete coverage of the Agility Talar Component

4.4.2.5   Clinical Outcomes of Third Generation Total Ankle Arthroplasty

a) B-P Mark II Total Ankle System (Deep Sulcus)[*]

The original Mark I design was modified to improve talar fixation and reduce the risk of bearing subluxation. The results of this modification are reported in:

> Buechel FF, Buechel FF. Jr., and Pappas MJ: Twenty Year Evaluation of Cementless Mobile-Bearing Total Ankle Replacements. *Clinical Orthop.* 424:19-26, 2004.

There were 74 patients (75 implants) Mark II B-P ankles implanted over a twelve-year time span. Using a strict ankle scoring system, the system had good/excellent results in 88% of the cases. Cumulative survivorship using an endpoint of revision of any component was 92%.

The authors concluded that mobile-bearings improve the success of total ankle replacement by minimizing wear and loosening problems [22].

"Considering the current status of ankle fusion and progressive hind foot arthritis known to follow, cementless, mobile-bearing ankle replacement, with the ability to exchange worn bearings if needed, offers a reasonable alternative in properly selected patients".

---

[*] Also see Ref. 37 Doets H.C.: 6 (2-13) Year Results with the LCS/Buechel-Pappas Mobile Bearing Prosthesis. ERASS ,2002.

Doets HC, Brand R., Nelissen R: Total Ankle Arthroplasty in Inflammatory Joint Disease: Five to Sixteen Year Results with Two Mobile –Bearing Designs *JBJS(Am)*,2006:88:1272-1286.

A two center observational study on results of 74 Mark II B-P ankles and 19 Mark I ankles. Mean 8-year overall survival was 83.6% (95% confidence interval). Wear or fracture of the polyethylene bearing did not occur.

The authors concluded mobile-bearing ankle replacement is a valid treatment option for the rheumatoid ankle if proper indications are applied. Aseptic loosening and persistent deformity were the most important modes of failure [54].

Su EP, Kahn B, and Figgie MP: Total Ankle Replacement in Patients with Rheumatoid Arthritis. *Clinical Orthop:* 424:32-38, 2004.

There were 19 patients (18 implants) implanted over a ten-year time span. Using a strict ankle scoring system, the system had good/excellent results in 79% of the cases. Cumulative survivorship using an endpoint of revision of any component was 95%.

The authors concluded that the early to intermediate results in patients with end-stage RA show that they are doing well. However, tibial osteolysis incidence warrants close follow up [53].

Keblish DJ et al: Eight Year of a minimally Constrained Total Ankle Arthroplasty, Unpublished 2005

There were 31 ankle prostheses were implanted in 23 patients between 1990 and 1997. 28 ankles in 21 patients were evaluated clinically and radiographically with an average follow up of 8.3 years.

The authors concluded that 'improvements in prosthetic design such as cementless fixation and decreased constraint appear to make total ankle arthroplasty a more predictable procedure.' They added that 'despite a variety of complications, we are encouraged by intermediate term results in a select low demand arthritic population' [36].

The study is summarized in Table 4.6 as follows:

Table 4.6 Clinical Data on the Buechel – Pappas Mark II Total Ankle Replacement.

Study	Buechel (33)	Doets (37)	Su (53)	Keblish (36)
Number of cases	75 (74 Patients)	74	19	31 (23 patients)
M/F	Male = 34 Female = 40	-	Male = 2 Female = 17	Male = 2 Female = 21
Age (mean)	49	58	50	61
Diagnosis	PTA=55 (73%) OA= 8 (11%) RA= 9 (12%) ON= 3 (4%)	RA= 74 (100%)	RA = 19(100%)	RA = 31 (100%)
Follow-up	Mean 5 Years	Mean 8 Years	Mean 5 Years	Mean 8.3 yrs (range 5-12 yrs)
Delayed Wound Healing	11 (15%)	7 (9.4%)	0 (0%)	4 (13%)
Talar Subsidence	3 (4.0%)	1 (4%)	0 (0%)	4 (13%)
Bearing subluxation	0 (0%)	0 (0%)	1 (5%)	0 (0%)
Severe bearing wear	3 (4%)	0 (0%)	0 (0%)	1 (3%)
Malleolar fracture	6 (6%)	-	0 (0%)	10 (32%)
Infection	2 (3%)	6 (8.1%)	1 (5%)	0 (0%)
Reflex sympathic Dystrophy	3 (4 %)	0 (0%)	0 (0%)	0 (0%)
Tibial component loosening	0 (0%)	3 (4%)	2 (11.5%)	3 (10%)
Survivorship (%)	92 (Kaplan-Meier) Revision for any reason at 12 yrs	89 Revision for any reason at 10 yrs	95 Revision for any reason at 6 years	93 Revision for any reason at 8 yrs
Average Overall Clinical Score (%)	88 (NJOHAEF)	77 (AOFAS)	81 (AOFAS)	81 (AOFAS)

From Ref. 22 it may be seen that talar subsidence is greatly reduced compared to the original design and that bearing subluxation was completely eliminated. The single case of severe bearing wear in Ref. 22 was the result of a tibial component malpositioning. In this case, only half of the bearing engaged the tibial component articulating surface plate. This mal-positioning produced significantly increased contact stresses and accelerated the bearing wear due to the metal edge of the plate wiping over the bearing during ankle motion.

San Giovanni et al. [55] in a study of the B-P Mark II in 31 ankles with an average follow up of 8.3 years obtained results quite similar to those of Ref. [22]. They report a survivorship of 93% and an 82% complete satisfaction rate and rated their tibial pain as mild to none. They also, however, report tibia or talar component subsidence as a potential problem in 18% of the patients.

Komistek et al [56] show that gait after a B-P Mark II replacement is essentially normal. That gait after arthrodesis is, as expected, abnormal as is shown by Wu et al [57].

In comparing the performance of the B-P ankle and the Agility, it should be noted that the mean age of Dr. Buechel's patients with a B-P ankle (Ref. 2) are significantly younger than in Dr. Alvine's patients (Refs [22] and [48]) being 49 and 63 years, respectively. The patient demographics and diagnoses are similar being 19% osteoarthritis and 12% rheumatoid arthritis, respectively.

b)   Additional References
Lewis [59], Saltzman [60, 61] and Alvine [48] review the state of the art of the S.T.A.R. ankle devices and find that they, with cautious use, have a place in ankle treatment. Wood et al [49] presents good results with the S.T.A.R. Saltzman et al in Ref. [62] describes the effect of the Agility device on ankle ligaments. Jung et al [63] propose the use of plating to reduce syndesmosis nonunion, common with the Agility device. Grisberg et al [64] describe and discuss revision of painful ankle fusion with an Agility ankle replacement and conclude it may be preferable to amputation of the foot. McGarvey et al [65] compare malleolar fractures in the S.T.A.R. and Agility devices, a significant complication in ankle replacement, and suggest means for its reduction and treatment.

Kobayashi et al [66] describe the nature of wear particles in knee and ankle replacements and find them similar. Of interest they find similar wear in the congruent S.T.A.R. and incongruent Agility devices. Nicholson et al [52] find that the contact stress of the incongruent Agility device is excessive at least for some patients.

Wood et al [67] compare a cemented incongruent ankle device with an uncemented congruent mobile bearing device and finds that the latter is far superior. Su et al [53] report on the generally successful application of the Mark II B-P device for the replacement of the ankle in rheumatoids. Bonnin et al [68], Hintermann et al [69] and Leardini et al [70] describe newer mobile bearing ankle devices that have demonstrated generally good performance.

4.4.2.6   Analysis of the Third Generation Total Ankle Designs

Although the performance of the B-P Mark II device is quite good for an ankle replacement further improvement is needed to approach the performance of a modern hip or knee. The two remaining problems that need addressing are those of excessive cyst formation and of talar subsidence. Additional development and research are needed to bring the level of performance of ankle devices to that of other modern prostheses.

4.4.3   Design of the B-P Ankle System

4.4.3.1   Design History

The authors' collaboration on ankle design began when they first met in 1974. Their first effort was the B-P Cylindrical Ankle Replacement shown in Fig. 4.16

[8]. Six such devices were implanted during 1974 and 1975. Failure due to loosening occurred in 5 of 6 devices within the first year. It was clear from the inspection of the retrieved specimens that this loosening was the result of the lack of axial rotation in the device. Further there was pitting on the UHMWPe talar component, likely caused by the edge effect [15].

The desire to allow axial rotation while providing a congruent articulation led the authors to develop a spherical articulation, based on the Smith Total Ankle [6]. This design is illustrated in Fig. 4.27.

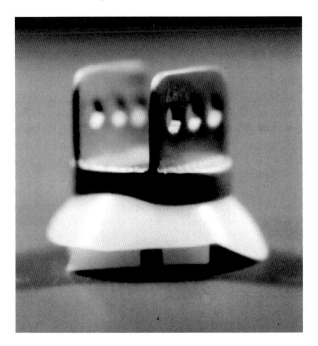

Fig. 4.27 B-P Spherical Total Ankle Replacement.

The edge effect noted in the cylindrical device was accommodated by "camming" the edge of the tibial articulation surface in the spherical device [71].

On analysis this design, unfortunately, had two serious weaknesses. First, it did not provide essentially total coverage of the resected tibia and talus. Secondly, and most importantly, it did not provide normal I-E stability. This latter problem is illustrated in Fig. 4.28.

This led to the introduction of a mobile bearing, first used by the authors in their "floating socket" shoulder prosthesis [16], to ankle devices. The result was the B-P Trunion Ankle Replacement of Fig. 4.17. It was implanted in two patients and did well clinically.

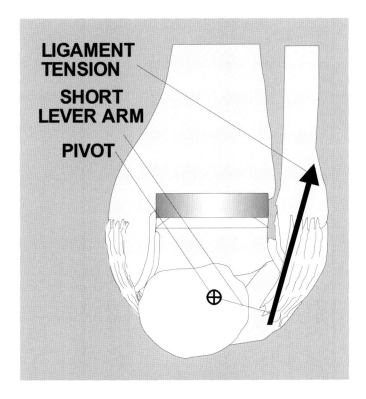

Fig. 4.28 Abnormal I-E Stability.

Although the performance of this device was satisfactory, as a result of the authors development of the LCS knee in 1978 [72], it occurred to them that a meniscal type bearing would eliminate unnecessary ML and AP constraints and thus provide a superior design. This lead to the development of the LCS, or B-P Mark I, Total Ankle Replacement device as illustrated in Fig. 4.18.

This design also worked reasonably well but due to the failures discussed earlier the Mark I design was changed in order to reduce blood supply disruption and risk of bearing subluxation. The result was a design with a deeper sulcus and shorter, dual fins. This dual fin arrangement also reduces the tendency of a fin to transfer load distally, thus reducing stress protection. Further, finite element analysis of the Mark I indicated that the tibial plate was too thin [73]. Its thickness was, therefore, increased in the Mark II.

This new design is more difficult to implant since it requires additional sculpture of the talus and another fin slot. The expected improved performance, however, outweighed this difficulty in the design decision to adapt the new configuration. The Mark II design is shown in Fig. 4.21. The differences between the Mark I and Mark II are illustrated in Fig. 4.29.

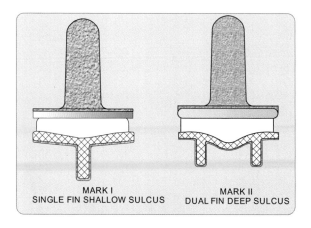

Fig. 4.29 Comparison of the Mark I and Mark II Devices.

The Mark II was developed in 1989. By this time the authors had also developed a ceramic coating which apparently provided greatly improved wear resistance, based on simulated wear tests [74], and enhanced biocompatibility [75].

The new design was successful in greatly reducing talar subsidence as illustrated by comparing the results given in Table 4.7 [22].

Based on the published literature, the B-P Mark II performed reasonably well in both short and long term clinical use. Although the rate of talar subsidence is well below that of the LCS Mark I Ankle it was felt, nevertheless, further improvement was possible. The B-P Mark III is an attempt to address the problems associated with the Mark II device.

Delayed wound healing was handled by the use of nasal oxygen for 48 hrs. Malleolar fracture was dealt with by improved instrumentation. Talar component subsidence and related severe bearing wear was treated by a change in the talar fixation by replacing the dual fins with dual pegs to further reduce disruption of the talar blood supply. Osteolysis was attacked by greatly improving the surface properties of the TiN coating. Although very little wear was observed in retrieved bearings where osteolysis was present, even this extremely low wear apparently can produce this condition.

Table 4.7 Complication in the B-P Mark I and Mark II Clinical Studies.

	LCS® Sliding Cylindrical Shallow-Sulcus TAR 40 cases 2 to 20 years F/U mean 12 years Ages: 21 to 89 mean 55		Buechel-Pappas® Deep-Sulcus TAR 75 cases 2 to 12 years F/U mean 5 years Ages: 25 to 78 mean 49	
Complications	**# of Ankles**	**%**	**# of Ankles**	**%**
Delayed Wound Healing	9	22.5	11	14.7
Talar Component Subsidence	6	15.0	3	4.0 *
Bearing Subluxation	4	10.0	0	0.0 *
Severe Bearing Wear	5	12.5	3	4.0 *
Malleolar Fracture	3	7.5	6	8.0
Infection	2	5.0	2	2.7
Reflex Sympathetic Dystrophy	2	5.0	3	4.0
Tibial Component Loosening	0	0.0	0	0.0
Osteolysis Tibia	2	5.0	6	8.0
Osteolysis Fibula	1	2.5	2	2.7
Osteolysis Talus	1	2.5	2	2.7

* Mechanical Improvements

These changed resulted in the B-P Mark III Total Ankle Replacement System shown in Fig. 4.30

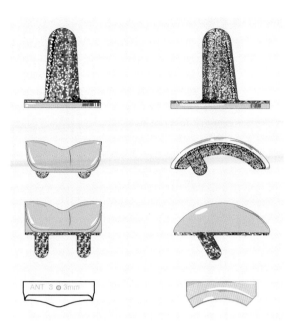

Fig. 4.30 B-P Mark III Total Ankle Replacement System.

and instruments shown in Fig. 4.31.

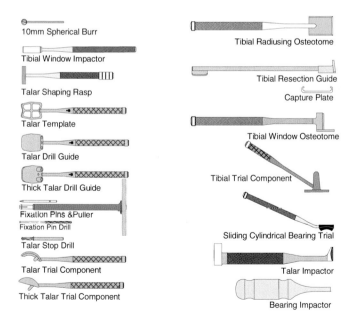

Fig. 4.31 B-P Mark III Total Ankle Replacement Instruments.

4.4.3.2 Properties of the B-P Mark III

a) Surfaces

The primary articulation of the Mark II and III are generated by the use of a generating curve, as shown in Fig. 4.32. It is similar to, but smaller than, that used to generate the articular surface of the New Jersey knee [72].

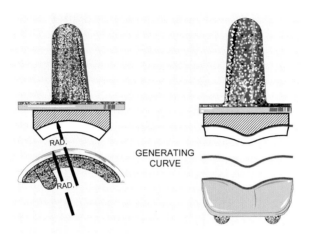

Fig. 4.32 Use of Common Generating Curve for the Talar and Bearing Articulating Surfaces.

In the ankle, however, since the range of motion is considerably less than the knee, a single talar radius of revolution is used rather than the multiple radii used in the knee. This single generating radius allows full congruity in the ankle for the entire motion range.

b) Ankle Motion

The B-P ankle provides near normal plantar and dorsiflexion well beyond the motion required for walking as illustrated in Fig. 4.33.

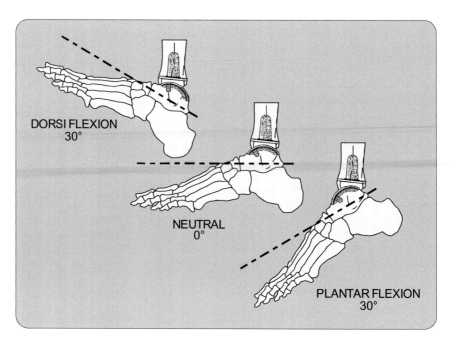

Fig. 4.33 B-P Ankle Maximum Plantar-Dorsiflexion.

It also provides unlimited axial rotation as illustrated in Fig. 4.34.

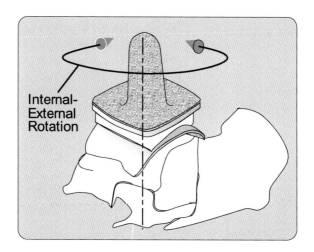

Fig. 4.34 Unconstrained Internal-External Rotation.

The B-P ankle also provides limited inversion-eversion of the tibiotalar joint without loss of congruity of the contact surfaces as shown in Fig. 4.35.

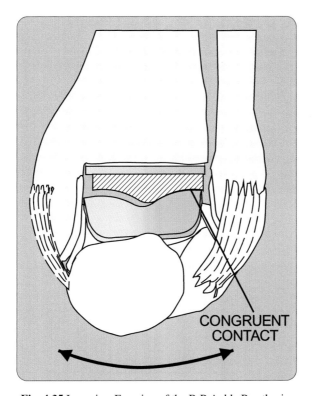

Fig. 4.35 Inversion-Eversion of the B-P Ankle Prosthesis.

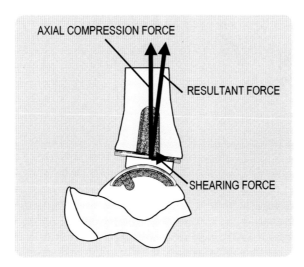

Fig. 4.36 Lateral View of the B-P Mark III Showing the Posterior Inclination of the Tibial Plate.

c) A-P Stability

The A-P stability of the B-P ankle is primarily extrinsic, as is the natural ankle. A seven degree posterior inclination of the tibial platform, as shown in Fig. 4.36, provides posterior shear resistance of about 0.12 times the joint reaction force or a maximum of about 0.6 times body weight. This is most of the estimated posterior shearing force and thus this force need not be taken by the ankle ligaments.

d) M-L and I-E Stability

Since the B-P Ankle resurfaces the tibiotalar joint with near natural articulating surfaces it is similar in these stability modes to the normal ankle as illustrated in Fig. 4.37.

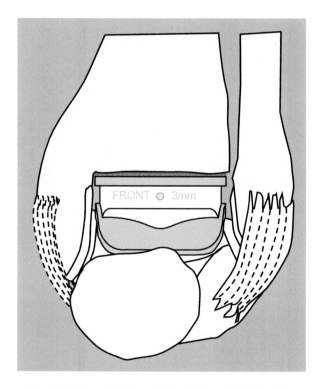

Fig. 4.37 Normal M-L and I-E stability of the B-P ankle.

e) Force Resistance

Equations, sufficient for use in knee and ankle prostheses, for the computation of the contact stress of two bodies in contact were developed in the 1930's [76]. These have been applied to the evaluation of knee and ankle prostheses [77, 78].

Since the B-P mobile ankle bearing allows both "Congruency and Mobility" just as does the NJ LCS knee bearing, the calculation of the contact stress in the B-P ankle articulation predicts low contact stress. This value computed at the maximum load given in [3] is appended to the results of the knee studies of Ref. [78] and is shown in Fig. 4.38.

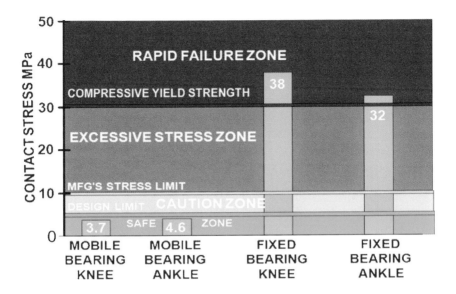

Fig. 4.38 Surface Contact Stress for the B-P Mark III Ankle and Typical Fixed Bearing Prostheses.

f) Wear
The low contact stress associated with the B-P ankle will produce less wear than the typical fixed bearing ankles that have performed badly. Still the estimated contact stress in the B-P ankle is somewhat higher than in the NJ LCS knee. Sliding motion in the ankle is, however, much less than in the knee, mitigating wear. It is desirable, nevertheless, to provide superior bearing surfaces for prosthetic ankle articulation. The authors have been developing a ceramic coated articulating surface since 1988. The first implantation's occurred in 1989. In its current form the surface is polished to a 0.5micro inch finish so as to minimize wear. Furthermore, the first author is currently using γ highly cross-linked UHMWPe in an effort to further reduce wear.

g) Fixation
The fixation of the B-P Mark III Ankle is illustrated in Fig. 4.39.

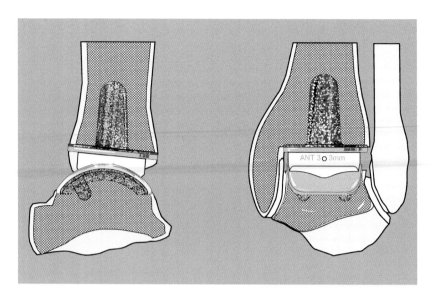

Fig. 4.39 Mark III B-P Ankle Fixation Geometry.

The dual Peg fixation of the talar component is used for the purpose of obtaining fixation on both sides of the talus while minimizing disruption of the talar blood supply. This is expected to minimize talar resorption and associated talar component tilt, encountered in the earlier single and dual fin designs. The primary blood supply of the talus is inferior and central to the talus [50]. The short, anterior, dual pegs minimize this disruption.

The short fixation peg of the tibial component is designed to help resist tilting forces on the tibia resulting from off-center loads. Early designs with a dual fin fixation were originally used and worked well in the relatively few cases of trunion ankles implanted. During 1977, analysis of meniscal bearing and rotating platform knee components indicated that the short, central stem provided superior fixation to fin fixation. Therefore, this concept was adapted to the ankle tibial fixation in 1978, abandoning the dual fin design of the original B-P tibial components. The author's long term, 30 year, experience with tibial knee components verifies the analysis of 1977. The fins of the bicruciate retaining tibial component normally show radiographic lucencies around the fins. These lucencies are rare with the posterior cruciate retaining tibial platform where off center loading of the tibial component is greater than in the bicruciate platform. Although loosening is not a significant problem with either design, radiological loosening is more apparent in the finned design.

The fixation surfaces are three-layer BioCoat® commercially pure titanium sintered bead porous coating on a titanium alloy substrate. The mean pore size is about 325 microns. The porous coating is itself covered with a coating of TiN ceramic.

4.4.4 Remaining Problems

4.4.4.1 Cysts

Wear particle disease known as osteolysis of bone has become a significant problem after total ankle replacement [79]. Fine polyethylene (UHMWPe) particles, often in the submicron range have been identified in tibial, talar and fibular cysts that begin to develop 3 to 4 years after surgery in a high percentage of patients who are sensitized to these particles. The blood supply to the ankle is more remote than the hip or knee making transport of the particles away from the ankle less likely. This would subject the ankle tissues to increasing concentrations of macrophages and giant cells laden with proteolytic enzymes.

These "osteolytic cysts" are usually painless and imperceptible to the patient and are only discovered by routine x-ray evaluation during the yearly follow-up examinations. If progression of cystic size is seen over a one to two year interval, a CT scan of the ankle is recommended to evaluate the location, volume and extent of the cysts. If they become expansile, a malleolar or talar fracture can occur, causing failure of the ankle replacement by subsidence or displacement of a malleolar fracture.

Treatment is directed at curettage and bone grafting of all cystic lesions greater than 1 cm. and replacing the polyethylene with a more durable and wear resistant bearing. In some cases, when the entire ankle and subtalar joints are extensively involved and ligamentous instability complicates the condition, a calcaneal-tibial fusion can be performed using an intramedullary rod and locking screws combined with extensive bone grafting of the large tibiotalar defects associated with prosthetic removal.

4.4.4.2 Talar Collapse

A catastrophic complication, seen occasionally, involves talar body collapse which can be secondary to avascular necrosis or progressive osteolysis.

a) Avascular Necrosis (AVN)
When the blood supply to the talus is interrupted by trauma or surgery, the body of the talus can undergo osteonecrosis and collapse. In this situation a talar component will subside into the avascular bone, become painful and often unstable.

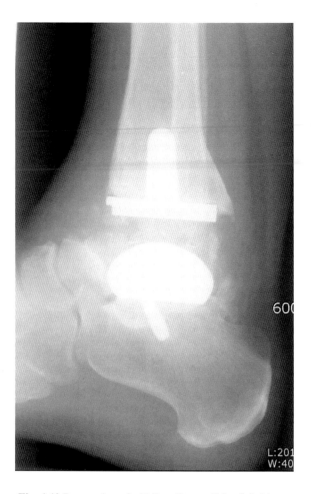

Fig. 4.40 Restoration of a Failure Due to Talar Subsidence.

b) Progressive Osteolysis

When the mechanism of osteolysis involves most of the talar body, the supporting bone can fail, just as in AVN. In both situations when the talar prosthesis has failed fixation and collapsed through the talar body, the talar component and osteolytic bone needs to be removed. A "custom talar body "prosthesis can be used to replace this severe bone loss. The 2 fixation stems of this device must use the calcaneus for bony anchorage and stability in such cases. If stability can be achieved with improved, wear resistant bearings, excellent function can be restored. However, if alignment and stability cannot be achieved with these custom implants, it is advisable to perform a calcaneal-tibial fusion for long term stability and function. An example of talar component subsidence and restoration with a "custom talar body" replacement is seen in Fig. 4.40.

4.4.5 The Future

Current ankle replacement design has narrowed down to mobile bearing, three part devices, mostly based on the original LCS design of 1978. These devices vary with regard to design details and materials. All seem to work well in the short and medium term except for problems associated with UHMWPe wear.

The major problem is the adverse reaction to even minor UHMWPe wear. These problems are manifest in cyst formation and bone necrosis which result in subsidence and loosening. Solutions to this problem appear to be better metallic surface finishing and bearing materials which are now under investigation and, hopefully, should provide a solution and elevate ankles to the same level of success seen in the more successful hip and knee replacements. After the wear problem is solved long term clinical experience may provide insight into the desirability of design features and materials in the different designs in clinical use.

4.5 Conclusion

Analysis, experimentation and clinical results clearly show the two piece, incongruent ankles have been incapable of providing a satisfactory ankle replacement. They have been discontinued most everywhere except in the United States of America where a reactionary FDA has discouraged the use of internationally accepted and successful three part designs for more than three decades.

Recently the quarter century old STAR ankle replacement has received FDA approval after a long and costly clinical trial. This should provide a better device than has been available in the USA. The introduction of more current mobile-bearing designs is still prohibited by the FDA. Thus, typically European manufacturers of mobile bearing designs introduce an inferior, fixed bearing version for sale in the USA.

The mobile bearing Mark III B-P Ankle is the culmination of more than thirty years of development. It fully exploits the mobile bearing concept by maintaining complete congruity for all phases of motion. Further it provides normal ankle motion and stability along with this congruity. The low wear ceramic coating of superior biocompatibility along with its porous coated ingrowth fixation geometry provide a realistic expectation for a long life and perhaps a lifetime joint replacement once the problems of cysts and talar collapse are resolved.

References

[1] Leardini, A., et al.: Mobility of the Human Ankle and the Design of Total Ankle Replacement. Clinical Orthop. 424, 39–46 (2004)
[2] Leardini, A., et al.: 0 Kinematics of the Human Ankle Complex in Passive Motion; A Single Degree of Freedom System. Journal of Biomechanics 32, 111–118 (1999)
[3] Stauffer, R.N., Chao, E.Y.S., Brewster, R.C.: Force and motion analysis of the normal, diseased and prosthetic ankle joint. In: Proceedings of the 23rd Annual Meeting of the ORS, Las Vegas Nevada, vol. 44 (1977)

[4]   Fitzgerald, E., Chao, E.Y.S., Hoffman, R.E.: Goniometric measurement of ankle motion A method for clinical evaluation. In: Proceedings of the 23rd Annual Meeting of the ORS, Las Vegas Nevada, vol. 43 (1977)

[5]   Stauffer, R.N., Chao, E.Y.S.: Torsional stability of the Mayo total ankle arthroplasty. In: Proceedings of the 25th Annual Meeting of the ORS, San Francisco, CA, vol. 112 (1979)

[6]   Dini, A.A., Bassett, F.H.: Evaluation of the early result of Smith total ankle replacement. Clin. Orthop. (146), 228–230 (1980)

[7]   Stauffer, R.N.: Total joint arthroplasty, The ankle. Mayo Clin. Proc. 54(9), 570–575 (1979)

[8]   Pappas, M., Bucchel, F.F., DePalma, A.F.: Cylindrical Total Ankle Joint Replacement: Surgical and Biomechanical Rationale. Clinical Orthopaedics and Related Research 118, 82–92 (1976)

[9]   Buechel, F.F.: Complications of 292 total ankle replacements. Presented at the Ninth Annual Meeting of the Foot and Ankle Society, San Francisco, CA (1979)

[10] Stauffer, R.N., Segal, N.M.: Total ankle arthroplasty: four years' experience. Clin. Orthop. 160, 217–221 (1981)

[11] Lachiewicz, P.F., Inglis, A.E., Ranawat, C.S.: Total ankle replacement in rheumatoid arthritis. J. Bone Joint Surg. Am. 66A(3), 340–343 (1984)

[12] Kitaoka, H.B., Patzer, G.L.: Clinical results of the Mayo total ankle arthroplasty. J. Bone Joint Surg. Am. 78A(11), 1658–1664 (1996)

[13] Unger, A.S., Inglis, A.E., Mow, C.S., Figgie, H.E.: Total ankle arthroplasty in rheumatoid arthritis: a long-term follow-up study. Foot and Ankle 8(4), 173–179 (1988)

[14] Kitaoka, H.B., et al.: Survivorship Analysis of the Mayo Total Ankle Arthroplasty. J. Bone Joint Surg. Am. 76A, 974–979 (1994)

[15] Buechel, F.F., Pappas, M.J.: Failure mode of cylindrical total ankle replacement. Presented at the Tenth Annual Meeting of the Foot and Ankle Society, Atlanta, GA (1980)

[16] Buechel, F.F., Pappas, M.J., DePalma, A.F.: Floating-Socket Total Shoulder Replacement; Anatomical, Biomechanical, and Surgical Rationale. Journal of Biomedical Materials Research 12(1), 89–114, 197 (1978)

[17] Buechel, F.F., Pappas, M.J.: The New Jersey Low-Contact Stress Ankle Replacement System: Biomechanical Rationale and Review of the First 23 Cementless Cases. Foot and Ankle, American Orthopedic Foot and Ankle Society 8(8), 279–290 (1988)

[18] Kofoed, H., et al.: Cylindrical cemented ankle arthroplasty: A prospective series with long-term follow-up. Foot & Ankle Int. 16, 474–478 (1995)

[19] Kofoed, H., Danborg, L.: Biological fixation of ankle arthroplasty. The Foot 5(1), 27–31 (1995)

[20] Knecht, S.I., et al.: The Agility Total Ankle Arthroplasty. J. Bone Joint Surg. Am. 86A(6), 1161–1171 (2004)

[21] Feldman, M.P.: Buechel-Pappas Total Ankle Prosthesis: Results in Patients 5 to 7 Years after Implantation. Clinics in Podiatric Medicine and Surgery 23(5), 733–743 (2006)

[22] Buechel, F.F., Buechel Jr., F.F., Pappas, M.J.: Twenty Year Evaluation of Cementless Mobile-Bearing Total Ankle Replacement. Clinical Orthop. 424, 19–26 (2004)

[23] Federal Register, Section 888.3110: 47/128:29070 (1982)

[24] Scholz, K.C.: Total ankle arthroplasty using biological fixation components compared to ankle arthrodesis. Orthopedics 10(1), 125–131 (1987)

[25] Waugh, T.R., Evanski, P.M., McMaster, W.C.: Irvine ankle arthroplasty. Prosthetic design and surgical technique. Clin. Orthop. 114, 180–184 (1976)

[26] Evanski, P.H., Waugh, T.R.: Management of arthritis of the ankle. An alternative of arthrodesis. Clin. Orthop. 122, 110–115 (1977)

[27] Wynn, A.H., et al.: Long-term Follow-up of Conaxial (Beck-Stefee) Total Ankle Arthroplasty. Foot and Ankle 13, 303–306 (1992)

[28] Jensen, N.C., Kroner, K.: Total ankle joint replacement: a clinical follow up. Orthopedics 15(2), 236–239 (1992)

[29] Herberts, P., Goldie, I.F., Korner, L., Larsson, U., Lindborg, G., Zachrisson, B.E.: Endoprosthetic arthroplasty of the ankle joint. A clinical and radiological follow-up. Acta Orthop. Scand. 53(4), 687–696 (1982)

[30] Helm, R., Stevens, J.: Long-term results of total ankle replacement. J. Arthroplasty 1(4), 271–277 (1986)

[31] Bolton-Maggs, B.G., Sudlow, R.A., Freeman, M.A.: Total ankle arthroplasty. A long-term review of the London Hospital experience. J. Bone Joint Surg. Br. 67B(5), 785–790 (1985)

[32] Takakura, Y., Tanaka, Y., Sugimoto, K., Tamai, S., Masuhara, K.: Ankle arthroplasty. A comparative study of cemented metal and uncemented ceramic prostheses. Clin. Orthop. 1(252), 209–216 (1990)

[33] Kofoed, H., Sorensen, T.S.: Ankle arthroplasty for rheumatoid arthritis and osteoarthritis: prospective long-term study of cemented replacements. J. Bone Joint Surg. Br. 80(2), 328–332 (1998)

[34] Neufeld, S.K., Lee, T.H.: Total Ankle Arthroplasty: Indications, Results, and Biomechanical Rationale. American Journal of Orthopedics, 593–602 (2000)

[35] Newton, S.E.: Total ankle arthroplasty – a four-year study. Presented at the 44th Annual Meeting of the American Academy of Orthopedic Surgeons, Las Vegas (1977)

[36] Keblish, D.J., et al.: Eight Year of a minimally Constrained Total Ankle Arthroplasty (2005) (unpublished)

[37] Doets, H.C.: 2-13 Year Results with the LCS/Buechel-Pappas Mobile Bearing Prosthesis. In: ERASS (2002)

[38] Doets, H.C.: The Low Contact Stress/Buechel-Pappas Total Ankle Prosthesis. In: Kofoed, H. (ed.) Current Status of Ankle Arthroplasty, ch. 6. Springer, Berlin (1998)

[39] San Giovanni, T., et al.: Long-term follow-up with second generation, cementless Total Ankle Replacement. In: Annual Meeting of the American Orthopedic Foot and Ankle Society, AOFAS (1999)

[40] Valderrabano, V., Hintermann, B., Dick, W.: Scandinavian Total Ankle Replacement. Clinical Orthop. 424, 47–56 (2004)

[41] Schernberg, F.: Current results of Ankle Arthroplasty – European Multi-center Study of Cementless Ankle Arthroplasty. In: Kofoed, H. (ed.) Current Status of Ankle Arthroplasty, ch.9. Springer, Berlin (1998)

[42] Kofoed, H.: Scandinavian Total Ankle Replacement (STAR). Clinical Orthop. 424, 73–79 (2004)

[43] Kofoed, H.: Ankle Arthroplasty: Indications, Alignment, Stability and Gain in Mobility. In: Kofoed, H. (ed.) Current Status of Ankle Arthroplasty, ch.4. Springer, Berlin (1998)

[44] Saltzman, C.L., Alvine, F.G.: The Agility Total Ankle Replacement. In: Instr. Course Lect. AAOS, vol. 51, pp. 129–133 (2002)

[45] Rippstein, P.F.: Clinical experiences with three different designs of ankle prostheses. Foot Ankle Clin. N Am. 7, 817–931 (2002)

[46] Pyevich, M.T., et al.: Total ankle arthroplasty: A unique design. J. Bone Joint Surg. Am. 80, 1410–1420 (1998)

[47] Spirt, A.A., et al.: Complications and Failure after Total Ankle Replacement. J. Bone Joint Surg. Am. 86A(6), 1172–1178 (2004)

[48] Alvine, F.: Long-term results lend support to ankle arthroplasty. Orthopedics Today, 8–9 (August 2003)

[49] Wood, P.L., Deakin, S.: Total ankle replacement. The results in 200 ankles. J. Bone Joint Surg. Br. 85B(3), 334–341 (2003)

[50] Mulfiner, G.L., Trueta, J.: The Blood Supply of the Talus. J. Bone Joint Surg. Am. 52A(b), 160–167 (1970)

[51] Hostalen, G.U.R.: Hoechst Aktiengesellschaft. Verkauf Kunstoffe, 6230 Frankfurt am Main 80, 22 (1982)

[52] Nicholson, J.J., et al.: Joint Contact Characteristics in Agility Total Ankle Arthroplasty. Clinical Orthop. 424, 125–129 (2004)

[53] Su, E.P., Kahn, B., Figgie, M.P.: Total Ankle Replacement in Patients with Rheumatoid Arthritis. Clinical Orthop. 424, 32–38 (2004)

[54] Doets, H.C., et al.: Total Ankle Arthroplasty in Inflammatory Joint Desease. J. Bone Joint Surg. Am. 86A, 1272–1286 (2006)

[55] San Giovanni, T., et al.: Eight Year Results of a Minimally Constrained Total Ankle Arthroplasty. Fool and Ankle International 27, 418–426 (2006)

[56] Komistek, R.D., et al.: A determination of ankle kinematics using fluoroscopy. Foot and Ankle International 21(4), 343–350 (2000)

[57] Wu, D.P.M., et al.: Gait Analysis After Ankle Arthrodesis. Gait Posture 11, 54–61 (2000)

[58] Knecht, S.I., et al.: The Agility Total Ankle Arthroplasty. J. Bone Joint Surg. Am. 86A(6), 1161–1171 (2004)

[59] Lewis, G.: Biomechanics of and Research Challenges in Uncemented Total Ankle Replacement. Clinical Orthop. 424, 89–97 (2004)

[60] Saltzman, C.L.: Total Ankle Arthroplasty: State of the art. In: Instr. Course Lect. AAOS, vol. 48, pp. 263–268 (1999)

[61] Saltzman, C.L.: Perspective on total ankle replacement. Foot Ankle Clin. 5(4), 761–775 (2000)

[62] Saltzman, C.L., et al.: The Effect of the Agility Prosthesis Misalignment on the Peri-Ankle Ligaments. Clinical Orthop. 424, 137–142 (2004)

[63] Jung, H.G., et al.: Radiographic and Biomechanical Support for Fibular Plating of the Agility Total Ankle. Clinical Orthop. 424, 118–124 (2004)

[64] Greisberg, J., et al.: Takedown of Ankle Fusion and Conversion to Total Ankle Replacement. Clinical Orthop. 424, 80–88 (2004)

[65] McGarvey, W.C., et al.: Malleolar Fracture after Total Ankle Arthroplasty. Clinical Orthop. 424, 104–110 (2004)

[66] Kobayashi, A., et al.: Ankle Arthroplasties Generate Wear Particles Similar to Knee Arthroplasties. Clinical Orthop. 424, 69–72 (2004)

[67] Wood, P.L.R., et al.: Clinical Comparison of two total ankle replacements. Foot and Ankle Int. 21(7), 546–550 (2000)

[68] Bonnin, M., et al.: Midterm Results of the Salto Total Ankle Prosthesis. Clinical Orthop. 424, 6–18 (2004)

[69] Hintermann, B., et al.: The HINTEGRA Ankle: Rationale and Short-Term Results of 122 Consecutive Ankles. Clinical Orthop. 424, 57–68 (2004)

[70] Leardini, et al.: Mobility of the Human Ankle and the Design of Total Ankle Replacement. Clinical Orthop. 424, 39–46 (2004)

[71] Deutschman, A.D., et al.: Roller Bearings. Section 9-2: Machine Design. Macmillan, New York (1975)

[72] Buechel, F.F., Pappas, M.J.: Long-term survivorship analysis of cruciate-sparing vs. cruciate sacrificing knee prostheses using meniscal bearings. Clinical Orthopaedics and Related Research 260, 162–169 (1990)

[73] Crowell, H.P.: Three Dimensional Finite Element Analysis of a Totsal Ankle Prosthesis. Dissertation. New Jersey Institute of Technology (1990)

[74] Pappas, M.J., Makris, G., Buechel, F.F.: Comparison of Wear of UHMWPe Cups Articulating with Co-Cr and TiN Coated Femoral Heads. In: Transactions of the 16th Annual Meeting of The Society for Biomaterials XIII (1990)

[75] Hayashi, K., Matsuguchi, N., Uenoyama, K., Kanemaru, T., Sugioka, Y.: Evaluation of metal implants coated with several types of ceramics as biomaterials. J. Soc. Biomat. 23, 1247–1259 (1989)

[76] Pappas, M.J., Makris, G., Buechel, F.F.: Contact stresses in metal-plastic total knee replacements: A theoretical and experimental study. Biomedical Engineering Technical Report (1986)

[77] Buechel, F.F., Buechel Jr, F.F., Pappas, M.J.: Ten-Year Evaluation of Cementless Meniscal Bearing Total Ankle Replacement. Foot and Ankle Int. 24(6), 462–472 (2003)

[78] Pappas, M.J., Makris, G., Buechel, F.F.: Evaluation of contact stress in metal-plastic knee replacements. In: Pizzoferrato, A., et al. (eds.) Biomaterials and Clinical Applications, pp. 259–264 (1987)

[79] Buechel, F.F.: Osteolysis after Total Ankle Arthroplasty. Presented at the 35th Annual OST Society Meeting, Bonaire NA (2009)

Chapter 5
The Hip

Abstract. This chapter describes the anatomy, pathology and hip replacements developed to treat pathological hip conditions. The history of four generations of hip replacement designs, their evaluation in light of the material in Chapters I and 2 and the clinical performance of these designs is presented. The first and second generations met with partial success and led the way to the development of improved designs. The third generations of designs work well. Current designs have added modularity to further improve the flexibility in the use of hip replacements. Also presented is the design of a fourth generation hip system using the principles of the first three chapters. The design process of Chapter 3 was used for the development of an improved version of the B-P hip system. The system includes conventional, modular and surface replacement elements. Ceramic coated titanium alloy is used for its metallic components. Except for the effects of UHMWPe wear clinical results are quite good. Wear is a problem common to all hip replacement systems using UHMWPe bearings. Use of highly cross-linked UHMWPe, fortunately, shows considerable potential for solving this problem. Ceramic on ceramic articulating devices show excellent long term performance. Metal on metal, although initially promising, has essentially been abandoned due to the adverse effects of metal ions released by wear.

5.1 Anatomy

The complex known as the hip joint consists of the femoral head and the acetabulum (Fig. 5.1), articulating to accommodate extension, flexion and rotational movements, similar to a "ball and socket" joint.

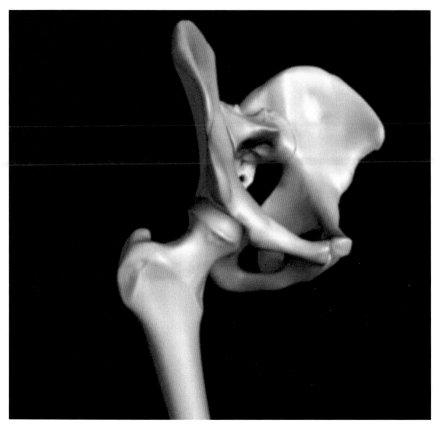

Fig. 5.1 The Hip Joint.

5.1.1 Ligamentous Structures

The ligamentous structures are integrated with the capsule to provide stability at the extremes of rotational motion. A transverse acetabular ligament maintains inferior acetabular stability of the anterior and posterior cotyledons of the "horseshoe-shaped" acetabular articular surface. A peripheral fibro-cartilaginous labrum provides added joint stability and helps to seal the synovial fluid film around the hip joint.

Additional stability is provided by the deep spherical acetabular socket that entraps the femoral head throughout its range of motion.

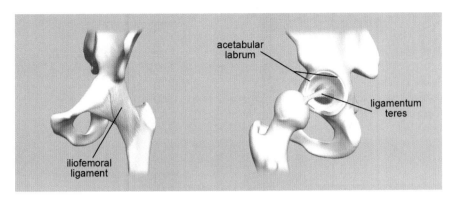

Fig. 5.2 Ligaments of the Hip.

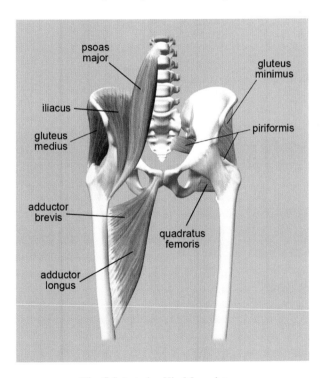

Fig. 5.3 Anterior Hip Musculature.

5.1.2 Musculature

The main muscles of abduction include the gluteus medius and gluteus minimus which originate from the lateral iliac wall and insert on the greater trochanter. They balance the pelvis during swing through of the gait cycle. The gluteus maximus provides hip extension while the iliopsoas, inserted on the lesser trochanter is the most powerful hip flexor.

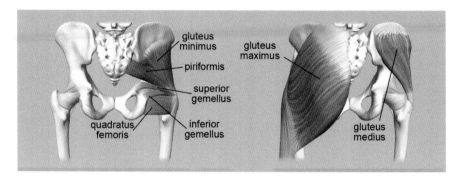

Fig. 5.4 Posterior Hip Musculature.

The pirifomis, gemelli and quadrates femoris muscles provide added posterior hip stability and act as short external rotators of the hip, while the adductor brevis, longus and magnus muscles provide adduction motion, while limiting unrestricted abduction.

The sartorius or "tailor's muscle" provides external hip rotation for crossing one leg over the other.

5.2 Biomechanics

5.2.1 Kinematics

Hip movement is simple three degree of freedom rotation, as illustrated in Fig. 5.5

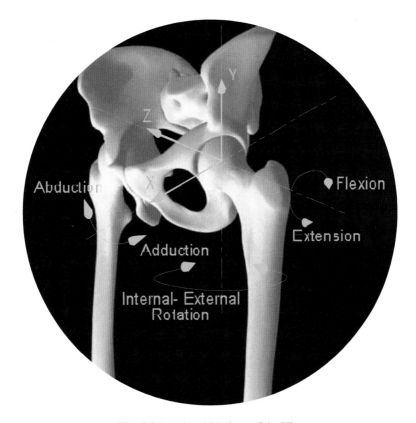

Fig. 5.5 Rotational Motions of the Hip.

The three rotatory degrees of freedom associated with the hip joint are:

1. Flexion - Extension; which is the principal motion of the joint.
2. Abduction – Adduction
3. Internal – External Rotation.

Normal mean range of motion (ROM) varies slightly, by about 3-5° with gender and race. Individual variations within groups are somewhat greater. The normal mean ROM in individuals in the 60 – 74 year age group (the most likely to have a hip replacement) is 118°(13° SD) flexion, 17°(8° SD) extension, 39°(12° SD) abduction, 30°(7° SD) internal rotation and 29°(9° SD) external rotation [1].

Any prosthetic restriction of this motion is undesirable as it may adversely affect hip function and can produce dislocation of a hip replacement. Thus, the surgeon should determine the ROM provided by the devices they implant and the ROM of their patients after implantation. Reliable and valid ROM measurement, however, requires great sophistication [2].

5.2.2 Stability

The hip is a stable ball and socket joint and, thus, is constrained against significant translation motion and unconstrained against rotary motion except as limited by adjacent tissue.

5.2.3 Forces

As in other load bearing joints, loads are cyclic and highly variable for different individuals and for different activities and phases of activities. Maximum compressive forces in the hip in relatively young normal males have been estimated to be on the order of five times body weight during normal walking [3, 4]. Other activities, such as stair ascent, are estimated to produce even higher values [4]. In vivo measurement [5, 6] of forces on the femoral head of patients with hip replacements, understandably, indicates much lower values on the order of half those estimated in Refs. [3, 4].

The direction of the force is also quite variable. In two legged stance, for example, the force vector is essentially vertical, In one legged stance, due to the balancing action of the abductors, the vector is inclined medially about 30°. Walking and other activities such as stair climbing and arising from a chair for example are more complex.

During level walking it is estimated that the vertical component of the force on the femoral head is about five times body weight, the A\P component about twice body weight acting anteriorly and the M\L component about equal to body weight acting medially [4].

Of particular interest is the observation of Paul [3] that the peak load vector on the femoral head is at an angle of about 148° to the femoral shaft. In a patient with a hip replacement the vertical force would be less than the values on which the 148° is based. In such patients, therefore, the shaft to neck angle would be larger since the adductor force, producing this angularity is less. Johnston and Brand [7] conclude that the optimum neck to stem angle is 150°.

5.3 Pathology

Disease processes involving the hip joint are usually classified into congenital, metabolic, neuro-muscular, infectious, autoimmune and post-traumatic.

5.3.1 Congenital

Incomplete or poor embryonic development of the hip can result from developmental dysplasia of the hip (DDH) or congenital dislocation of the hip (CDH) which involves poor femoral head coverage by the developing acetabulum, resulting in reduced acetabular depth and femoral head instability, leading to growth disturbances and earlier hip joint degeneration. Abduction bracing and acetabular osteotomies to improve head coverage are essential non-joint replacement procedures to improve these conditions.

5.3.2 Metabolic

Bone disorders involving deficiencies in calcium metabolism secondary to hormonal, genetic or nutritional imbalance can affect the integrity of the bones and ligaments of the hip, leading to joint destruction or malalignment. Additionally, vascular compromise of the femoral head thorough avascular necrosis (AVN) can destroy the hip joint articulation. Such disorders need to be accurately diagnosed and treated with medical or surgical management to avoid complete hip joint destruction.

5.3.3 Neuromuscular

Diseases affecting the nerves and muscles of the hip can cause significant gait disturbances and instability problems. Lumbar disc disease can have a disabling effect on the abductor function, while piriformis compression of the sciatic nerve can cause incapacitating pain and sciatic nerve related motor weakness. Cerebral palsy can affect hip adductors and cause contractures that lead to poor gait function and difficult personal hygiene. Such conditions require careful medical and non-implant surgical management to regain maximum function.

5.3.4 Infectious

Sepsis of the hip from any gram positive or gram negative bacteria can result in destruction of the hip joint, known as septic arthritis. These joints are at a significant risk of re-infection, but hip fusion is so disabling that multiple attempts at curing an infection using antibiotic impregnated bone cement is often attempted, even when abductor function is less than ideal. Ambulating with an "abductor lurch" seems to be preferable to a "stiff hip". Hip fusion, resection arthroplasty or suppressive antibiotic therapies are last resort options for persistent hip joint infections.

5.3.5 Autoimmune

Arthritis of the hip can be a result of autoimmune disorders such as rheumatoid or psoriatic arthritis, where the body perceives a foreign antigen to be present, requiring neutralization by host defenses, even though they are not foreign, but in fact, are the normal cartilage structure of the host. In the normal defense process, the host destroys its own normal cartilage by mistake. Evidence suggests that osteoarthritis has a genetic component that may be related to an autoimmune phenomenon as well. In any event, these arthritic conditions have a similar end-stage pathology, which makes them suitable candidates for joint replacement to improve their function.

5.3.6   Post-Traumatic

Fractures, dislocations or femoroacetabular impingement [8-12] can compromise hip joint function and in many cases cause severe cartilage destruction, similar to osteoarthritis. In patients with progressive joint destruction despite anatomic alignment of fractures or removal of impinging FAI cam/pincer lesions, hip joint replacement offers an excellent functional alternative to disabling pain, stiffness and deformity. An x-ray of post-traumatic hip arthritis is seen in Fig. 5.6.

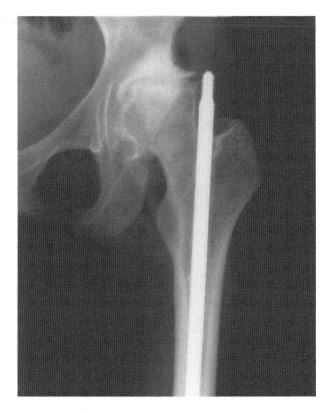

Fig. 5.6 Post Traumatic Hip Arthritis.

5.4   HIP Replacement

5.4.1   Design Evolution

5.4.1.1   Early Arthroplasty

Interposition, or mold, arthroplasty was first performed by several surgeons during the 19th century using human and animal tissue. The limited use of metal interposition was introduced and used in the late 19th and early 20th centuries with limited success [13]. However, it was not until Smith-Peterson introduced the use of a glass interposition cup in 1923 that the door was cracked open to successful prosthetic arthroplasty of the hip [14].

Total hip replacement was attempted by Gluck [15] late in the 19th century using ivory components and much later, in about 1958, by Wiles [16] who used a metal ball and socket device. The unavailability of appropriate materials and a lack of understanding of mechanical design and biomechanics combined with a lack of understanding of the fixation prevented the development of successful total joint replacement in these early attempts.

5.4.1.2 First Generation Designs – Interposition Cups

a) The Smith-Peterson Cup

Smith-Peterson continued to refine his design by use of several different materials [17]. He finally chose a new high temperature resistant alloy developed for gas turbine use for his device. This metal, made by Howmet, a developer and manufacturer of exotic metals is a Co-Cr-Mo alloy, which they called "Vitallium". It is now the most common metal alloy used for orthopaedic implants.

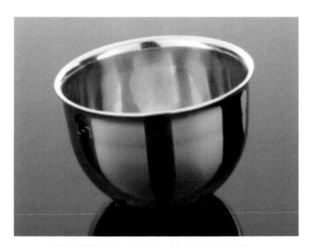

Fig. 5.7 Smith- Peterson Interposition Cup.

b) Acetabular Interposition Cups
The Smith-Petersen type interposition cups were intended to articulate with the acetabulum. Urist [18] and McBride [19], in the late 1950's, introduced inter-position cups for essentially resurfacing the acetabulum. These designs are the precursors of the acetabular cups used in total hip replacement. The McBride cup is shown in Fig. 5.8.

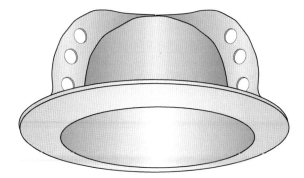

Fig. 5.8 McBride Interposition Cup.

5.4.1.3 Second Generation Designs – Hemi Replacements

The limited success and applicability of interposition arthroplasty made the development of improved devices highly desirable. The next series of designs focused on femoral head (hemi) replacements as a means of improvement.

a) The Judet Surface Replacement
A variation of the Smith-Petersen approach was used by the Judet brothers [20] from about 1946 wherein the cup used a central stem to augment fixation. They originally used an acrylic head but due to excessive wear they ultimately moved to Co-Cr-Mo heads. These devices where the precursors of the femoral head resurfacing devices used today.

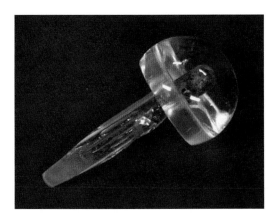

Fig. 5.9 Judet Femoral Components.

b) Austin-Moore
Austin-Moore introduced the concepts of fixing a head replacement with an intramedulary straight stem by press fit into the femoral shaft. The proximal

section of the stem was fenestrated in the hope that ingrowth would help stabilize the implant [21]. Several variations of this concept were developed and are still sold today for hemi replacement but fixtured by cement rather than press fit.

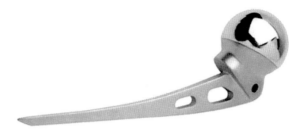

Fig. 5.10 Austin-Moore Femoral Component.

c)   The Thomson Femoral Component
The Thomson femoral component used a shorter curved stem [22].

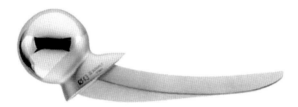

Fig. 5.11 Thompson Femoral Component.

d)   Others
Many variations of the designs of Austin-Moore and Thompson were introduced and are still available today.

5.4.1.4   Third Generation Designs – Total Replacements

The next logical step in the evolution of hip arthroplasty was additional attempts at the development of a total hip replacement based on the knowledge gained from the relative success of hemi arthroplasty. Hundreds of designs emerged in the 1970's. Discussed here are some of the important examples.

a)   The McKee-Farrar Total Hip Replacement
The need for a total hip replacement led first to the development of devices such as the McKee-Farrar total hip replacement which used a variation of the Thompson femoral stem and an acetabular interposition cup [23].

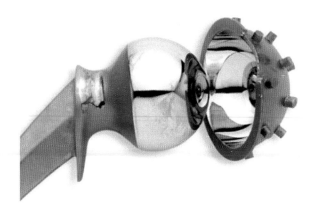

Fig. 5.12 The McKee-Farrar Total Hip Replacement.

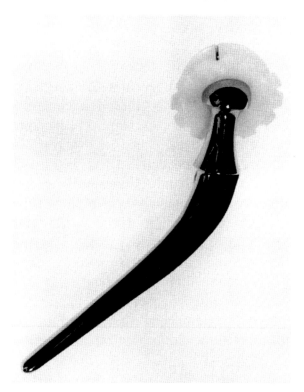

Fig. 5.13 The Charnley Total Hip Replacement.

b) The Charnley Cemented Total Hip Replacement

The breakthrough in the development of truly successful hip replacement came though the work of John Charnley [24, 25].

He worked with engineers to develop both an acetabular component capable of providing satisfactory wear resistance combined with the application of a biocompatible grouting agent of adequate strength to provide relatively stable fixation of the prosthesis components to bone.

c) The Müller Total Hip Replacement

Many variations of the Charnley followed. Perhaps the most widely accepted was the Müller device in its myriad forms. One of these are shown in Fig. 5.14 [26, 27].

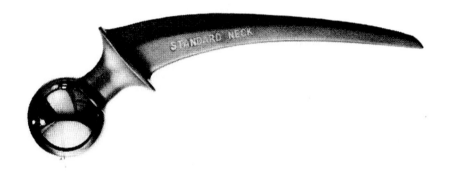

Fig. 5.14 Müller Hip Stems.

d) The Ring total Hip Replacement

Ring felt it was best to avoid cement and, thus, persisted with a screw augmented press fit design [28].

e) The Bipolar Acetabular Cup

Acetabular cups of the third generation were typically all UHMWPe and fixtured by use of cement. Acetal (DuPont Delrin) cups were investigated but abandoned due to DuPont's refusal to sell its Delrin to orthopaedic manufacturers for implant use. This was a wise decision in light of the potential toxicity of Delrin wear products.

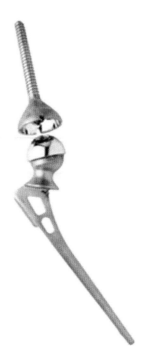

Fig. 5.15 The Ring Total Hip Replacement.

Acetabular degeneration and protrusion associated with monoblock Austin-Moore or the Thompson type femoral head replacement led developers to seek alternate solutions. One was total hip development. The other was a "Bipolar" hip replacement. In this latter concept a movable femoral head is used to reduce the amount of sliding articulation with the acetabulum by providing articulation between the head and stem of the femoral component. Such an approach was first proposed by Bateman [29] and then later by Christensen [30] and Gilberty [31]. In the Gilberty prosthesis the Bipolar Acetabular cup consisted of a metal, highly polished, outer shell and an UHMWPe liner. It was intended for use with the total hip femoral stems of the time.

Pappas and Buechel [32] introduced the concept of "Positive Eccentricity", used in the "Universal Self-Aligning Acetabular Component", which allowed more predictable positioning of the cup on the stem and improved function. This effect is illustrated in Fig. 5.16.

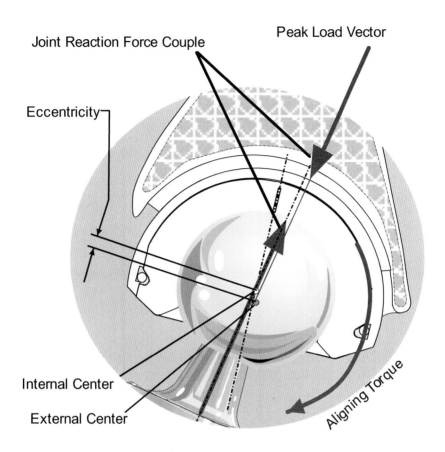

Fig. 5.16 Effect of Positive Eccentricity.

The Universal Self-Aligning Acetabular Component is kept aligned with the load vector by the effect of the Positive Eccentricity built into the bearing insert. The outside spherical surface of the bearing is made eccentric to the inside surface by an amount given by the equations in Ref. [32]. Such eccentricity produces a small force couple when the cup is not aligned with a joint load vector. Since the effect is greatest when a misalignment exists with the peak load vector, the cup tends to align itself with this vector. Such alignment ensures that the cup edge does not wipe across the articular cartilage and that contact always occurs with the spherical portion of the cup [32].

When the Universal Self-Aligning cup is used with the Buechel-Pappas Femoral Stem, the cup opening becomes centered on the femoral stem neck. This maximizes the motion possible between the cup and neck before impingement occurs, thus maximizing the range of motion of the components, reducing motion between the metal cup and acetabulum, and thereby reducing acetabular erosion.

f) Ceramic-on-Ceramic
Boutin introduced ceramic-on-ceramic articulation total hip replacement in the early 1970's [33]. These devices utilized both cemented and press fit acetabular components and a ceramic head on a femoral stem [34]. Ceramic surfaces are hard, wear resistant and, most importantly, their wear products have much lower toxicity than UHMWPe or metal wear particles [35].

Such devices have been used in Europe for more than three decades. The overall performance of ceramic-on-ceramic total hips seems superior to metal-on-plastic or metal-on-metal devices [36] although there have been problems with acetabular loosening [37], ceramic fracture [38] and squeaking [39]. Reports of such problems have delayed the use of such devices in the United States until recently.

g) Surface Replacement
Several resurfacing total hip replacement designs were developed and used in the late 1960's and the 1970's [40-44]. In general, they were unsuccessful and abandoned by most [13].

5.4.1.5 Fourth Generation Designs – Biological Fixation and Femoral Head Modularity

Although bone cement proved to be an effective fixation media it did have limitations as discussed in Chapter 1. Problems with cement led to another attempt at press fit and biological fixation hoped for by earlier developers. These later attempts by Judet et al [45] and Lord et al [46] first used fixation surfaces with relatively large mm size beads and fully coated stems. Later developments led to the use of small, sintered bead [47] or plasma sprayed [48] fibrous layered porous coating on femoral stems and acetabular cups.

Further, the number of different stem sizes and neck lengths and other variations needed to treat the patient's size variations and pathologies in the patient populations treated was a serious inventory problem for hospitals and manufacturers. Modular femoral heads were introduced to provide some relief by making available heads which could be configured to produce different neck lengths. Further, modular heads reduced manufacturing cost by making the heads much easier to polish.

Again, as in the second generation cemented total hips, a large variety of porous coated femoral stems and metal backed acetabular components were introduced into the orthopaedic market place. Samples of the more important variations are given below:

a) Femoral Stems
It is much easier to prepare the femoral shaft for a decent press fit needed for biological fixation if the stem is straight. Thus, most of the successful designs, such as the AML shown in Fig. 5.17, used a straight stem.

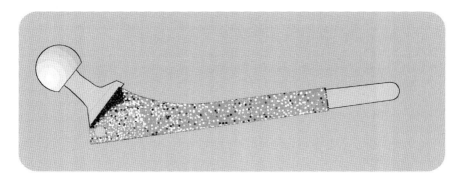

Fig. 5.17 The AML Porous Coated Femoral Component.

The Harris – Gelante [48] stem was titanium alloy with a sintered fiber-metal porous coating. It also used a calcar collar intended for load transfer to the femoral shaft through the calcar.

The AML [50] stem was made of Co-Cr-Mo alloy covered with a sintered bead porous coating. Initially it was fully coated with a relatively small bead of about 150µm. This was later changed to use a larger bead of about 325µm and the coating was removed from the end of the stem. The AML also uses a calcar collar.

The PCA used a Co-Cr-Mo proximally coated, stem with a relatively large sintered bead coating of about 500µm. The stem was available in different lengths as well as different stem diameters. The PCA stem was quite different from the HG or AML in that it used a doubly curved stem, which seems to make an accurate press fit almost impossible. Further it did not use a calcar collar but relied on diaphyseal fixation.

Femoral head modularity also allowed the successful development of ceramic heads for articulation with both ceramic or UHMWPe plastic lined acetabular cups. The heads were attached to the stems by means of a standard internal head and external stem tapers which allowed interchangeability of heads and stems across different manufacturers. Heads of various diameters such as 22, 26, 28 and 32mm became widely available.

b) Acetabular Cups

To avoid the use of cement a press fit acetabular component was required. This requirement implied the use of a metal backed UHMWPe acetabular component. Early efforts by Mittlemeir [51] and Lord et al [52] at metal backed screw in cups introduced in the 1970's, although initially accepted by some surgeons, were abandoned for porous coated cups by the early 1980's. Several variations were tried but the orthopaedic community finally settled on a hemispherical, porous coated, metal backed cup augmented by screws [53] or short pegs. More recently unaugmented hemispherical, porous coated metal backed cups have found acceptance due to problems with the use of augmentation screws [54].

c) *Resurfacing*

Notwithstanding the failure of metal to metal articulations in total hips McMinn has developed an apparently successful metal-to metal resurfacing prosthesis [55]. The elevated levels of metal ions in the blood are, however, of concern [56, 57] and thus, metal-to-metal articulation has been largely abandoned.

5.4.1.6   Fifth Generation Designs - Refinement

By the mid 1980's the second and third generation devices were working quite well. The major task was to await the long term results to allow an evaluation of competing concepts such as calcar vs. diaphyseal loading and the various articulation couples such as metal-plastic, ceramic- plastic, ceramic-ceramic and, in the case of surface replacement, metal-metal.

Improved material, manufacturing techniques and knowledge, however, also provide opportunity for design refinement, if not a major breakthrough. The Buechel-Pappas Hip Replacement System [58] is the result of refinement efforts based on such new knowledge and developments as shown in Fig. 5.18.

Optimized femoral stem and proximal porous coating geometries to reduce stress shielding and minimize thigh pain were developed [59].

Thin-film ceramic surface coatings have also been recently developed and mechanically tested for surface integrity and wear resistance [60-63].   These surfaces, when properly treated, offer significant improvements in wear resistance when used for articulation with UHMWPe [61]. When used to cover an entire porous coated prosthesis, the coating greatly reduces the surface exposure of the prosthesis thus avoiding increased metal ion release without preventing bone ingrowth. In addition, thin-film ceramic coating on a relatively soft substrate like titanium $(TiAl_6V_4)$ alloy hardens the surface against scratching from bone or third body abrasive particles, thus extending the use of titanium alloys for orthopaedic implant fixation without the risks of surface abrasion and metallosis [64].

Recently a potential solution to the primary remaining problem, excessive wear, is being introduced into the current designs. The development of highly cross-linked UHMWPe of 1.5.2.1 appears to substantially reduce wear in metal to plastic articulations.

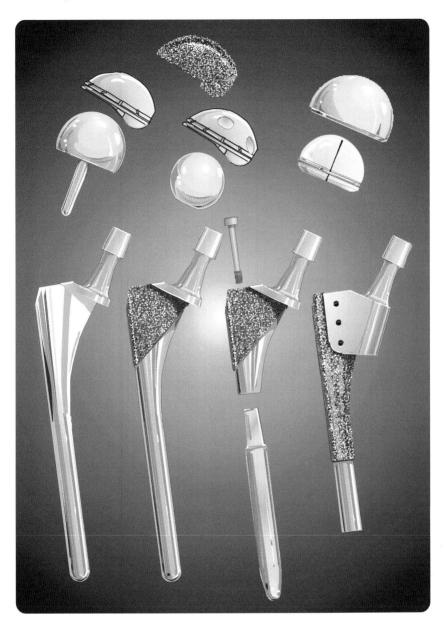

Fig. 5.18 The Buechel-Pappas Hip Replacement System.

5.4.2   Evaluation

5.4.2.1   Clinical Outcome of First Generation Hip Arthroplasty

These interposition arthroplasty designs were of limited usefulness in that they could not treat most hip pathology. Where they were useful pain reduction was partial at best and there were long term problems of erosion and protrusion. Although there were many cases of long term success with such devices, most resulted in ultimate failure. Relying upon simple femoral head coverage, though attractive early on, did not suit the needs of the surgeon involved in complex arthritic hip reconstruction. The unpredictability and persistent pain following cup arthroplasty, even with an added straight (Judet) or curved (Townley) central alignment stem, led surgeons away from uncemented femoral surface "caps" to more dependable intramedullary stems.

5.4.2.2   Clinical Outcome of Second Generation Hip Arthroplasty

Hemiarthroplasty broadened the range of treatable pathologies of the hip and improved somewhat on the performance of the first generation. The essential problems of the first generation, pain, acetabular erosion and protrusio, although reduced, still persisted. Thus, as in the case of the first generation although there were many cases of long term success with such devices, many resulted in ultimate failure. Persistent or progressive "groin pain", experienced by many patients, led surgeons to explore alternative options that would reduce or eliminate this disabling condition. The best course of action was to explore concepts that would resurface or replace the acetabular side of the hip as well as the femoral side, to eliminate the nerve endings associated with pain in the entire hip joint, not just the femur.

5.4.2.3   Clinical Outcome and Analysis of Third Generation Hip Arthroplasty

a)   The McKee-Farrar Total Hip Replacement
Early results with the press fit device were generally unsatisfactory [13, 21-23]. Later use was with cement which produced improved results but the design fell out of favor due to the availability of the superior Charnley device.

b)   The Charnley Cemented Total Hip Replacement
This device became, in essence, the gold standard. It is still widely used today more than a half century after its introduction. Although an excellent design for its time it, nevertheless, had design shortcomings.

The primary weakness is in the size of the femoral head. Although Charnley's group determined the optimal head size to be 22mm [25] this estimate was based on measurement of retrieved bearing wear of the various sizes of a stainless steel heads articulating against Teflon a slippery but not a good load bearing material. These results have little bearing on the articulating materials used a few years later.

Later investigation and testing by Weightman et al [65] of MIT found that the linear wear in a 22mm heads was 100% greater than with 32mm heads. Thus, wear penetration due to wear was substantially greater. Further, penetration due to creep is greater due to the higher stress associated with the smaller head. This penetration exacerbated the primary effect of the femoral head size and increased risk of hip dislocation.

c) The Müller Total Hip Replacement
The Müller device used a 32mm head which was preferred by many surgeons due to its superior dislocation resistance and its apparent lower wear. Its clinical performance was comparable to that of the Charnley and it was widely accepted for a time. It is still in use today.

d) The Ring total Hip Replacement
The Ring Prosthesis initially suffered from the same problems as the McKee-Farrar and, thus was later used with cement. Further, the problems associated with metal to metal articulation, even where Co-Cr-Mo alloy was used, led to the use of an UHMWPe acetabulum. The Ring design, however, did not make sense as a cemented device and thus fell from favor.

e) The Bipolar Acetabular Cup
Problems with dislocation and separation plagued the early designs [66-72]. Design concepts addressing these problems are described later. These concepts were apparently successful.

f) Ceramic-on-Ceramic
The problems encountered with ceramic-on-ceramic hips appear to be primarily design related. Acetabular cup loosening [34], cup impingement [73, 74] and squeaking [75, 76] are all a function of hip replacement design and surgical technique. The application of the principles discussed later should result in devices which take full advantage of the superior wear and biocompatibility of ceramic-on ceramic articulation [77].

g) Surface Replacement
With the possible exception of the McMinn device, results with this generation of resurfacing devices were generally unsatisfactory primarily due to acetabular migration and loosening [13]. This problem appears to be the result of design deficiencies which required over reaming of the acetabulum.

5.4.2.4 Clinical Outcome and Analysis of Fourth Generation Hip Arthroplasty

a) Femoral Stems
Cementless total hip replacement researchers, while recognizing the long-term benefits of fixation and function [79], have identified proximal femoral stress shielding as a growing concern for extensively porous-coated prostheses [80, 81]. Attempts to reduce proximal stress shielding by limiting the amount of bone

ingrowth to the proximal region of the femoral component have met with limited success in that specific design configurations both with and without calcar loading collars have produced an unsatisfactory level of thigh pain [58, 82-85]. Additionally, osteolysis, femoral component subsidence and lack of proximal fixation have lessened the appeal for this approach [86-88].

The Harris – Galante stem became collarless after it was found that even only proximal porous coating produced stress shielding of the collar and good diaphyseal fixation was obtainable without a collar. Short term results, however, still seemed inferior to a well fixed cemented implant [13, 50].

Initially the AML was unsatisfactory due to excessive femoral stress shielding by fixation at the tip [85]. Removal of the porous coating from the tip of the stem helped since torsion of the femoral shaft inhibited distal fixation. When the tip was coated such torsion produced little micro motion allowing fixation to occur. Today the AML is widely used with good clinical results [89, 90] comparable to that of the Charnley hip [91].

The Porous Coated Anatomic (PCA) went through a number of minor changes, particularly a reduction in the amount of bowing, in an attempt to make implantation practical. It never, however, achieved clinical success [92].

Diaphyseal, rather than calcar loading, with proximal sintered bead porous coating has become the principal means of load transfer to the femoral shaft. The rationale for this is that it was found that even with only proximal coating there was substantial calcar resorption. Thus, the collar had little purpose. Further, it was felt, by some, that the collar might interfere with diaphyseal loading [13].

b) Acetabular Cups
The Mittelmeir and Lord screw-in cups, although accepted initially by orthopedists, were quickly abandoned due to a multitude of problems. These included; excessive bulk requiring excessive bone removal, difficulty in orientation and inadequate fixation leading to neck – to - cup impingement, dislocations, cup loosening and migration [13].

Similarly, cementless, hemispherical acetabular components with stable polyethylene bearing liners have been evaluated [93] and used clinically with good mid-term success after 5 to 10 years [59, 94]. The industry finally settled on a Harris – Gelante type hemispherical cup fixtured by sintered bead porous coating usually with adjunctive screws and/or pegs. This type produced good clinical results and is used even in an uncoated form with cement.

5.4.2.5 Clinical Outcome and Analysis of Fifth Generation Hip Arthroplasty

It is of interest to evaluate the use of a fifth generation totally cementless modular total hip replacement, which uses a straight-stemmed femoral component with optimized proximal porous coating and an anatomically shaped, hemispherical acetabular cup. The metallic components are coated with titanium-nitride-ceramic to reduce wear on the bearing surfaces, to minimize ion leaching from the porous coated surfaces and to provide abrasion resistance for the femoral stem.

Clinical, radiographic and implant survivorship are compared to standard long-term cemented and cementless hip replacements results to establish the impact of this new technology.

a) Material and Methods
From April 30, 1990 to March 31, 1999 there were 141 hip replacements implanted into 127 patients. Eleven hips in 10 patients were excluded from analysis because 2 were lost to follow-up immediately post operatively and the remaining 8 patients expired before the two-year examination. Of the 130 hips in 117 patients available for examination with a minimum two year follow up, twenty hips in 10 patients died at an average of 6.3 years after surgery (2.2 to 10.8 years), all with well functioning implants, and one was lost to follow-up at 4.6 years after surgery. Methods to locate all patients were exhausted using the following methods: internet yellow page search, social-security death index search, social security TRW commissioned search firms, last known phone number/relative contacts, referring or covering physician contacts, and hospital/clinic contacts. The patient demographics and diagnoses of minimum two year surviving patients are noted in Table 5.1.

Table 5.1 Patient Demographics.

		130 hips in 117 patients	
1. DIAGNOSIS			
Osteoarthritis		103	
Post-traumatic arthritis		6	
Rheumatoid arthritis		10	
Avascular necrosis		11	
Gender			
Male		52	
Female		78	
	RANGE	**AVERAGE**	
Height (Inches)	58-76	65.7	
Weight (pounds)	90-300	180.2	
Age (at Surgery)	30.5-90.2	66.3	

All implants used in this study were cementless devices (Buechel-Pappas™ Integrated Total Hip Replacement System, Endotec, Inc. Orlando, Florida). The titanium alloy ($TiAl_6V_4$) acetabular cup is hemispherical with inferior extensions and an anatomical inferior cut-out (Fig. 5.18).
Cups were available with no, or five spherically seated, holes for screw fixation, passed through the metallic shell which was porous-coated on its outer surface with sintered commercially pure titanium beads to give an average pore size of 350 microns and a volume porosity of 30% (BioCoat®, Endotec, Inc.). Titanium alloy ($TiAl_6V_4$) 6.5 mm cancellous bone screws (Endotec, Inc.) were

used in varying sizes to stabilize the acetabular cup in 17 hips. In the remaining 114 hips, the acetabular cup was press-fit without screws using a 1 mm interference fit for hard bone such as in osteoarthritis and a 2 mm interference fit for soft bone such as in rheumatoid arthritis. A flexible lipped UHMWPe bearing liner is snapped into recessed grooves in the metal shell to complete the assembly. The original design (Mark I) bearing contained several of these flexible lips. A design change was made in 1994 to increase the number of these lips to the full circumference of the bearing (Mark II) to provide more fixation to the metal shell. Acetabular defects were curetted and bone grafted with autologous femoral head as needed.

The titanium alloy femoral component was of a straight-stemmed, proportional size configuration with an optimized proximal porous coating under the 30° angled collar, on the anterior and posterior surfaces as well as the lateral surface of the component.

The femoral head was made of titanium alloy coated with a polished 6 to 10 micron thick layer of titanium-nitride-ceramic (TiN) (UltraCoat®, Endotec, Inc.) applied by means of a proprietary, physical vapor deposition (PVD) process. The entire femoral stem and porous coated regions were also coated with UltraCoat, TiN.

Pre and post-operative clinical evaluations were performed on all patients using the Harris Hip rating Scale [95]. Radiographic analyses were performed using the technique of DeLee and Charnley [96] for assessing acetabular radiolucency and the method of Drucker et al [97] for measuring cup migration. The femoral component was evaluated for radiolucencies by the method of Gruen et al. [98] and for stress shielding of the calcar by the method of Hamlin et al [59]. Mechanical complications, clinical complications and mechanisms of failure were recorded and analyzed.

Kaplan-Meier Survival Analysis [99] was performed using endpoints of revision of any component for any reason, a clinically poor hip score or radiographic evidence of failure (radiolucency of over 2 mm in all zones surrounding an implant) or gross implant migration.

b) Result
Pre-operative Harris Hip Scores averaged 46, range 22 to 74. Post-operative Harris Hip Scores averaged 93, range 64 to 100. In patients with over 2 year follow-up, average 6.43, range 2.25 to 11.2 years (130 hips in 117 patients) there were 107 (81.7%) excellent, 20 (16%) good, 3 (2.3%) fair and 0(0%) poor results noted.

Temporary thigh pain graded as mild and not interfering with activities of daily living was seen in 6 out of 130 hips (4.6 %) and moderate in 1 out of 130 (0.8%). Mild thigh pain resolved at an average of 2.1 years; moderate thigh pain associated with a traumatic trochanteric fracture resolved after 3.2 years.

1) Radiographic Analysis - Acetabular Cup
Radiolucencies around the acetabular cup remained stable over time with no cup migrations noted, (Table 5.2). One component was revised elsewhere for reported

Table 5.2 Acetabular Component Lucencies (Average lucencies in millimeters).

	1 Yr.	2 Yr.	3 Yr.	4 Yr.	5 Yr.	6 Yr.	7 Yr.	8 Yr.	9 Yr.	10 Yr.
	Interval	Interval	Interval	Interval	Interval	Interval	Interval	Interval	Interval	Interval
ZONE	(n=130)	(n=99)	(n=77)	(n=59)	(n=47)	(n=33)	(n=23)	(n=17)	(n=9)	(n=4)
1	0.022	0.015	0.032	0.017	0.060	0.088	0.135	0.018	0.089	0.275
2	0.023	0.015	0.006	0.075	0.023	0.070	0.065	0.018	0.000	0.050
3	0.023	0.041	0.149	0.122	0.091	0.055	0.043	0.147	0.278	0.000

loosening, but radiographs were not available for examination prior to or since revision despite contact with the revising surgeon.

2) *Radiographic Analysis - Femoral Stem*

Radiolucencies of less than 1 mm were seen around the femoral stem tip in zones 4 on the AP and lateral views at the 2 year interval in 75% of cases but did not correlate with thigh pain. Zone 3 and 5 on AP and lateral views demonstrated radiolucencies less than 1 mm in approximately 50% of cases, (Table 5.3 and 5.4).

Table 5.3 A-P Femoral Lucencies (Average Lucencies in millimeters).

	1 Yr.	2 Yr.	3 Yr.	4 Yr.	5 Yr.	6 Yr.	7 Yr.	8 Yr.	9 Yr.	10 Yr.
	Interval	Interval	Interval	Interval	Interval	Interval	Interval	Interval	Interval	Interval
ZONE	(n=130)	(n=99)	(n=77)	(n=59)	(n=47)	(n=33)	(n=23)	(n=17)	(n=9)	(n=4)
1	0.010	0.069	0.058	0.161	0.096	0.048	0.122	0.000	0.000	0.000
2	0.003	0.010	0.021	0.102	0.021	0.039	0.022	0.018	0.033	0.000
3	0.015	0.048	0.142	0.168	0.079	0.206	0.317	0.224	0.222	0.125
4	0.066	0.342	0.408	0.366	0.402	0.642	0.570	0.482	0.611	0.750
5	0.052	0.124	0.129	0.231	0.123	0.182	0.174	0.176	0.256	0.200
6	0.007	0.010	0.045	0.183	0.085	0.070	0.043	0.088	0.167	0.000
7	0.010	0.010	0.003	0.090	0.021	0.021	0.043	0.000	0.000	0.000

Calcar atrophy [59] was minor, being rated as type 1 in 10% of cases reviewed (90 hips), type 2 in 5.6%, and type 3b in 1.1 %

No cases were severe enough to be in the Engh Type II calcar stress shielding category, which is a marked improvement over the AML prosthesis, which demonstrated 36 out of 381 hips (9%) with Engh type II stress shielding [79]. The worst case of calcar resorption in this study was in the Engh type I stress shielding category.

Table 5.4 Lateral Femoral Lucencies (Average Lucencies in millimeters).

	1 Yr. Interval (n=130)	2 Yr. Interval (n=99)	3 Yr. Interval (n=77)	4 Yr. Interval (n=59)	5 Yr. Interval (n=47)	6 Yr. Interval (n=33)	7 Yr. Interval (n=23)	8 Yr. Interval (n=17)	9 Yr. Interval (n=9)	10 Yr. Interval (n=4)
ZONE										
1	0.000	0.045	0.029	0.047	0.079	0.006	0.052	0.012	0.000	0.000
2	0.000	0.013	0.019	0.029	0.000	0.030	0.000	0.000	0.111	0.000
3	0.025	0.111	0.182	0.166	0.204	0.388	0.474	0.118	0.500	0.250
4	0.073	0.367	0.383	0.386	0.391	0.630	0.652	0.253	0.700	0.625
5	0.028	0.090	0.117	0.120	0.155	0.161	0.165	0.059	0.278	0.125
6	0.010	0.005	0.030	0.031	0.096	0.045	0.087	0.000	0.089	0.000
7	0.010	0.015	0.000	0.000	0.085	0.000	0.057	0.000	0.000	0.000

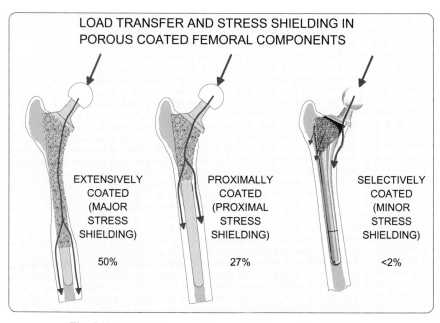

Fig. 5.19 Effect of Degree of Porous Coating on Stress Shielding

3) Mechanical Failures and Management

Two Mark I bearing liners dissociated from the acetabular shell after 4.8 and 6.8 years in an active 53 year old osteoarthritic male and in an active 77 year old osteoarthritic female. Both were replaced with Mark II bearing liners and both patients resumed normal activities without revising the well fixed acetabular components.

4) *Major or Minor Complications*

Complications experienced in this study are listed in Table 5.5.

Table 5.5 Complications Occurring in 130 Buechel-Pappas Primary Hips in 117 Patients.

COMPLICATION	Number	%
Peroneal Palsy	5	3.8
Permanent	1	0.8
Partial Recovery	1	0.8
Complete Recovery	3	2.3
Wound Dehiscence, Drainage	2	1.5
Trochanteric Bursitis, chronic	1	0.8
Thigh Pain	7	5.4
Mild	6	4.6
Moderate	1	0.8
Abductor Pain	1	0.8
Dislocation, all causes	4	3.1
Femoral Stem Loosening	0	0.0
Trochanteric fracture, traumatic	1	0.8
Sciatica	4	3.1
Acetabular Cup Loosening	1	0.8
Acetabular Bearing Dissociation	2	1.5
Periprosthetic Fracture	1	0.8
Femoral Stem Subsidence	1	0.8
Thrombophlebitis	1	0.8
Deep Venous Thrombosis	2	1.5
Heel decubitis ulcer	0	0.0
Hematoma, requiring evacuation	1	0.8
Lesser trochanter fracture, traumatic	1	0.8
Pes Bursitis	1	0.8
Pulmonary Embolism, non-fatal	2	1.5
Deep Infection	0	0.0

5) *Survivorship Analysis*

Kaplan-Meier [99] Survivorship analysis was performed using several end points:

1.   Revision of any component for any reason.
2.   Poor Harris Hip Score.
3.   Radiographic loosening or clinical loosening of any component.

These analyses are shown in Figs. (5.20- 5.22 respectively).

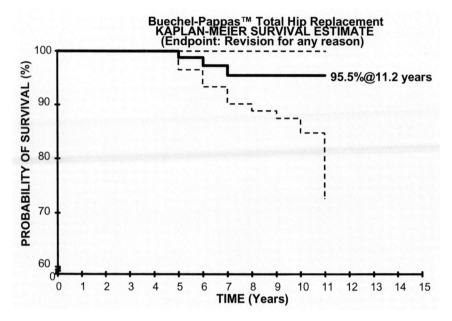

Fig. 5.20 Kaplan-Myer Survivorship of Buechel-Pappas Total Hip Replacements with and endpoint of revision for any reason.

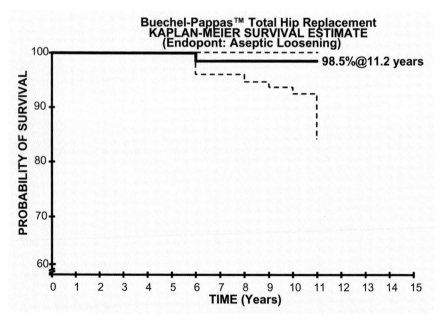

Fig. 5.21 Kaplan-Myer Survivorship of Buechel-Pappas Total Hip Replacements with and endpoint of a poor Harris Hip Score.

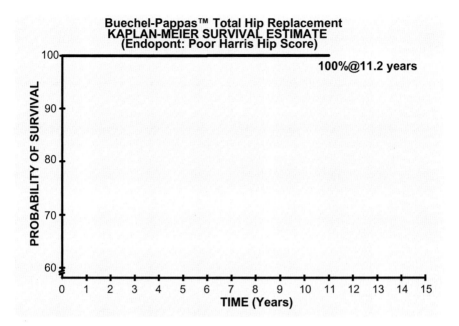

Fig. 5.22 Kaplan-Myer Survivorship of Buechel-Pappas Total Hip Replacements with and endpoint of aseptic loosening of any component.

c) Discussion

Long-term fixation and function, together with excellent wear resistance are the prerequisites for successful total hip arthroplasty. Survivorship analysis, radiographic analysis and clinical results are important outcome parameters by which orthopedic surgeons can measure the success or failure of one hip replacement system over another when used in similar patient populations. Primary hip replacement represents the best clinical condition to evaluate a new or improved prosthesis since the variables of major bone stock deficiencies associated with revision conditions are minimized or eliminated by study design. In this study there were 130 primary total hip replacements in 117 patients with minimum two year follow-up.

The femoral components used in this study were developed in response to the potential stress shielding problem posed by the extensively coated AML device developed by Emmett Lunceford in the late 1970's [59].

The femoral components were clinically developed to improve proximal femoral loading strain by means of a 30° angled loading collar and removing porous coating from the proximal medial region [59]. It has been shown by retrieval analysis that proximal medial bone ingrowth into a porous surface causes stress shielding even though the coating has been removed from the distal end of the stem [100]. This finding suggests that removal of the medial proximal porous coating and retention of anterior, posterior and lateral porous coating represents an ideal ingrowth configuration for maintaining stability while minimizing stress shielding. Finite element analysis of this improved stem and coating geometry concurs with the clinical observations [101].

Hemispherical, porous-coated acetabular cups have demonstrated excellent mid-term and long-term stability [58, 88]. Their use in total hip arthroplasty may represent a fixation improvement over cemented components [102]. However, premature wear, bearing dissociation and osteolysis have been reported with some of these devices [103-105] which casts some doubt as to whether these new devices are really improvements over the cemented Charnley acetabular cup which has documented superior survivorship [106]. Recent analysis of the acetabular cup geometries of currently available cementless devices has revealed that the optimal polyethylene liner geometry which maintains spherically-congruent articulation with the metallic acetabular shell has not been universally adopted [93].

The acetabular cup used in this study utilizes the spherically congruent-articulating-connection principles for the assembled cup and bearing liner [59]. This articulation has demonstrated superior stability and satisfactory wear resistance when articulated with polished titanium-nitride-ceramic femoral components in reciprocal, high-cycle simulation [61]. The current study provides clinical evidence to support the stability and durability of this cementless hemispherical acetabular component in vivo. One metallic acetabular cup was removed for reported loosening, and two Mark I (incomplete flexible lips) bearing liners were replaced (1.5%) after traumatic dissociation from the metallic cup. This represents an improvement over the Harris-Galante II acetabular component, which has a reported bearing liner dissociation of 2.6% in one study [105]. No Mark II bearing liners (complete flexible lips) were seen to dissociate from the metal cups.

The one acetabular cup that was revised elsewhere due to reported loosening of the acetabular component occurred 5.3 years after surgery. To date the authors have not been able to review the radiographs or obtain specific reasons for the revision with the caveat that the femoral stem was solidly fixed and retained.

The radiographic findings in the current study document the qualitative improvement in proximal bone density and lack of calcar atrophy with selective proximal porous coating over extensively coated devices. Engh et al [80] reported results showing that the amount of bone resorption was clearly related to the extent of the porous coating. One third coated stems have an incidence of 12.1% second or third degree bone resorption, two thirds was 33% and fully coated resulted in 54.3% of cases. These findings concur with a similar study in which the optimal femoral component was made of $TiAl_6V_4$ alloy [59] and used a similar proximal porous coating geometry. Further quantification of the actual bone density using DEXA scanning would be most helpful and should be considered as a future research direction.

Osteolysis around acetabular or femoral components was not seen. Radiolucent zones were non-progressive and less than 2 mm in Gruen zones 1 through 14. Femoral stem subsidence was encountered in 1 patient (0.8%), but was asymptomatic. No acetabular cup migration was encountered, although 1 (0.8%) acetabular component was revised elsewhere for reported loosening.

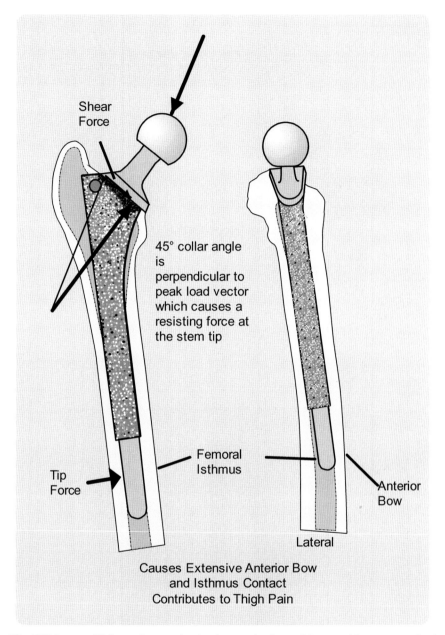

Fig. 5.23 Long, stiff femoral stems that impinge at the femoral bow, and have non-optimal 45° loading collars contribute to thigh pain.

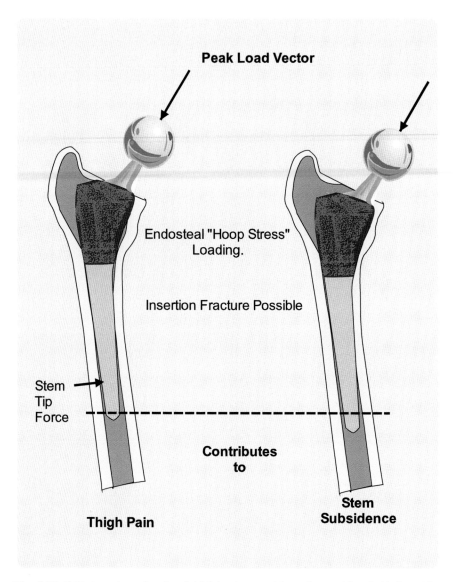

Fig. 5.24 Collarless stem showing initial implant position, along with subsided position contributing to thigh pain.

The clinical results of this study compare favorably to the long term results of the cemented [102, 107-109] and extensively coated cementless hip replacements [110, 111, 113]. They are superior to the reported results of other cementless proximally porous ingrowth devices [114-118]. Temporary thigh pain was noted in 7 patients overall. In 6 patients (4.6%) thigh pain was mild, did not interfere with activities of daily living. This pain resolved at an average of 2.1 years (range

2 to 6 years) after surgery. In one patient (0.8%) thigh pain was moderate and associated with chronic trochanteric bursitis following a greater trochanter fracture. This patient's pain resolved after 3.2 years. This was a significant improvement over other cementless devices [119, 120].

The mechanisms or causes of prosthetic thigh pain are multifactoral. Aside from long femoral stems that impinge at the femoral bow, suboptimal calcar loading occurs when a 45° angle collar is used (Fig. 5.23).

Since it is not perpendicular to the peak load vector, a shear force is developed which is resisted by a stem tip force that increases the lateral endosteal load and contributes to thigh pain. Collarless, circumferential, proximal porous coating stems have random subsidence and laterally displaced stem tip force may combine to cause thigh pain or uncontrolled leg length shortening (Fig. 5.24).

Campbell et al [120] reported a 22% incidence in thigh pain, which he attributed to these phenomena, along with bead shedding and distal periosteal reaction.

Post-operative dislocation was observed in 4 patients at 2 to 6 months post-op (mean 3.8 months). One dislocation was traumatic secondary to a fall. The other 3 dislocations occurred by excessive hyperflexion and internal rotation. All dislocations were successfully managed by closed reduction and brace immobilization for 6 weeks. The mean Harris Hip score for this group was 98 points (range 92-100).

Peroneal nerve palsy was encountered in the immediate post-operative period in 5 patients. In 3 patients full recovery was achieved after a mean of 1.4 years (range 1 to 2 years). Once patient had a partial recovery after 2 years but underwent a posterior tibial tendon transfer to improve her gait. One patient developed a permanent foot drop. No intraoperative complications were noted in any of these patients, but all implants were inserted through a posterior approach. The mean Harris Hip Score for this group was 85.8 points (range 65 to 96).

Kaplan-Meier survivorship analysis using an end-point of revision of any component for any reason was 95.5% at 11.2 years, which compares most favorably with the cemented Charnley and the cementless AML prostheses at the same time interval (Fig. 5.25).

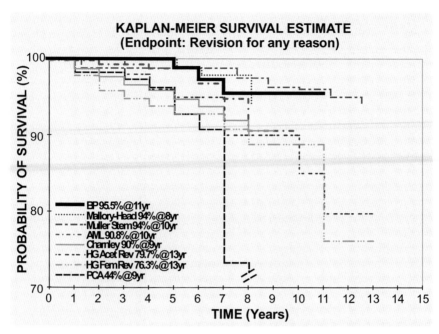

Fig. 5.25 Comparison of survival of Typical Third, Fourth and Fifth Generation Total Hip Arthroplasties.

The current prosthesis also improves upon the survivorship of the Mallory Head [117] (94% at 8 years), the Harris-Galante [113] (acetabular survivorship of 79.7% at 13 years and femoral stem survivorship of 76.3% at 13 years), and the PCA stem [116] (44% at 9yr).

Early clinical and survivorship results which document equivalence or superiority to standard devices while providing an improved feature, such as calcar retention, has been proposed as a method for improving joint replacement technology without sacrificing safety and efficacy [121]. The current study follows these guidelines for improving the state-of-the-art. Based on the current radiographic, clinical and survivorship data this proximally-porous-coated hip replacement offers design improvements over other standard devices and its continued use is recommended.

The refinements discussed in the next section produced outstanding results [58] with one exception, excessive wear. Time will tell if the use of ceramic-ceramic articulation or highly cross-linked UHMWPe will solve this remaining problem.

d) Resurfacing
The B-P resurfacing, notwithstanding the excellent simulator performance, did not fare as well clinically. Several wear throughs of the bearing were observed. They were easily revised by replacing the bearing liner. Still the problem of wear exists and additional work is needed to solve it.

5.4.3 Design of the B-P Hip System

Development of the Buechel – Pappas (B-P) Hip System began in 1982 and by 1985 had evolved into a straight stem, sintered bead, proximally porous coated, partial hemisphere metal backed acetabular cup, with screw fixation augmentation and a spherical resurfacing femoral head replacement using the same acetabular outer shell as used with the femoral stems. Initially Co-Cr-Mo was used for the metallic elements. They were in effect typical third generation devices.

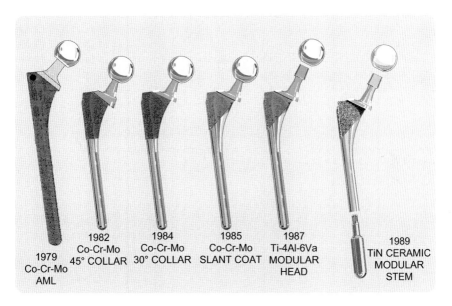

Fig. 5.26 Evolution of Proximally Porous Coated Femoral Components for Hip Joint Replacement.

A technical, manufacturing breakthrough led to the development of the fifth generation version. The economical casting of the metallic components in titanium alloy became practical. Thus, one could use the superior properties of titanium for the next generation device. Titanium is superior to the Co-Cr-Mo alloys in implant use in all important respects except abrasion resistance. To overcome this defect the B-P Hip System now employs a ceramic TiN coating which produces a surface hardness and abrasion resistance far superior to Co-Cr-Mo. This superiority is of particular importance for the metallic articulating surfaces since degradation due to the articulation is greatly reduced leading to the potential for wear reduction in long term use [122]. Further, tests [60], including a 48 million hip simulation test [61] showed greatly reduced wear in a TiN – UHMWPe articulating couple indicating the potential solution to the problems of excessive wear.

5.4.3.1 The Femoral Stem Components

a) Neck Alignment

The line of action of the joint reaction force vector varies with activity and phase. During the peak load phase of normal walking the vector is at an angle of about 148° [3] to the axis of the stem. This phase produces the highest stresses and loads in the femoral component and bone during walking.

A femoral shaft to neck angle of about 135° is optimal for the human femur, producing compressive stresses in the neck at peak loads with a bias medially for transfer of load through the calcar to the femoral shaft. This angle is not, however, optimal for a metal prosthetic neck. With the neck diameters used for femoral stems, this neck angle produces tensile stress in the lateral side of the neck which can lead to fatigue failure and increases the compressive stress in the medial side of the neck. Thus, neck diameters of 12mm and greater are typically used with 135° angle necks.

The B-P Femoral Stem System positions the head at the normal head location but medializes the distal neck junction to achieve a neck to stem angle of 148°, as shown in Fig. 5.27, thereby aligning the neck with the peak load vector. A neck diameter of 9mm is used. This smaller diameter neck and the neck – to - stem angle allow a greater range of motion than systems with a 12mm neck and 135° neck – to - stem angle.

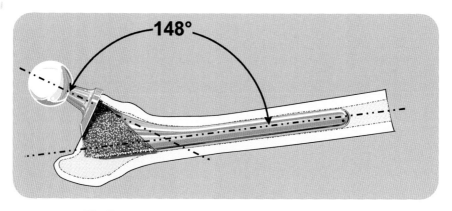

Fig. 5.27 The Buechel-Pappas Femoral Stem to Neck Angle.

This alignment eliminates tensile stresses and minimizes compressive stresses in the neck at this critical loading phase as illustrated in Fig. 5.28. This allows the safe use of a much smaller diameter neck providing an increased range of motion reducing the potential for impingement and dislocation.

Changing effective neck length by use of modular heads does not alter joint biomechanics during this phase as illustrated in Fig. 5.29.

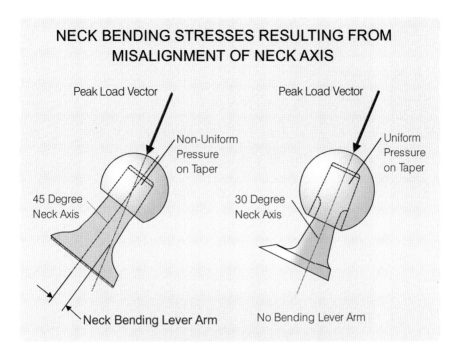

Fig. 5.28 Reduction of Neck Stress.

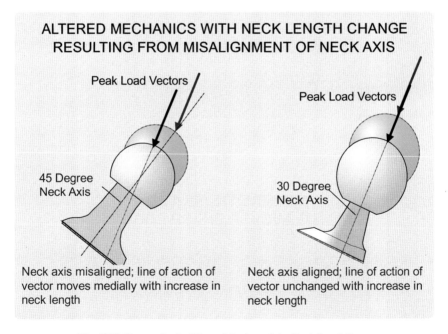

Fig. 5.29 Change in the Line of Action of the Peak Load Force.

Bipolar cups with positive eccentricity become aligned with the neck maximizing the effective ROM of the device as illustrated in Fig. 5.16.

b) Head Truncation

Integral femoral heads are often truncated for manufacturing convenience since it is easier to grind and polish truncated heads. Unfortunately, such truncation reduces the spherical surface available to resist bipolar cup dislocation and can introduce undesirable stress risers in the UHMWPe bearing thereby increasing wear and the possibility of pitting the bearing surface. It is interesting to note that modular heads are easier to manufacture than fixed heads and need not be truncated for ease of manufacture.

Current machining, grinding and polishing processes allow maintenance of the maximum amount of spherical surface avoiding problems associated with truncation and providing maximum resistance against bipolar cup separation. Thus, the B-P head is truncated only by the need for the conical cavity in the head as shown in Fig. 5.30.

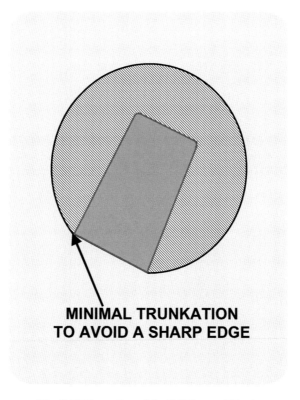

**MINIMAL TRUNKATION
TO AVOID A SHARP EDGE**

Fig. 5.30 Truncation of the B-P Femoral Head.

The reduction in the risk associated with excessive stress in the acetabular bearing is illustrated in Fig. 5.31.

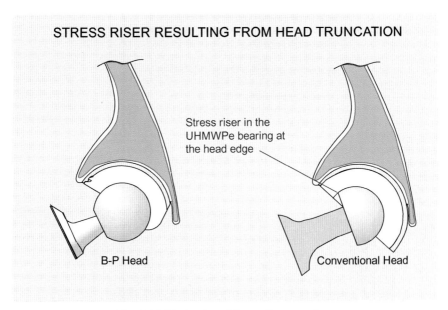

Fig. 5.31 Elimination of Stress Concentration.

The improvement in reducing the risk of Bipolar cup separation is illustrated in Fig. 5.32.

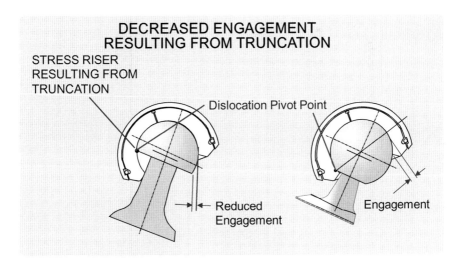

Fig. 5.32 Improvement in Separation Resistance.

c) *Collar Angle*

The reaction force acting on the collar is equal and opposite of the peak load vector. Since the collar on the B-P Femoral Stem is also perpendicular to the peak load vector, it is therefore perpendicular to the reaction force vector. Thus, a non perpendicular force component (shear force) is not needed to achieve a force balance and the collar-calcar interface is free of shearing force for the peak load phase.

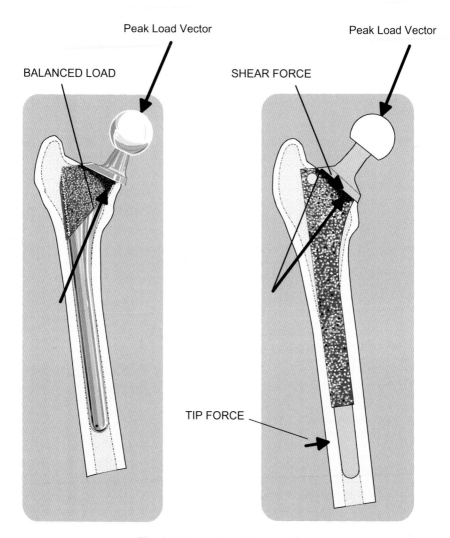

Fig. 5.33 Reduction of Shearing Forces.

Where the collar is at 45° to the shaft, and thus is not perpendicular to the peak load vector, a component parallel to the collar contact surface must exist in addition to a perpendicular reaction force component on this surface. Such a collar introduces undesirable shear at the collar-calcar interface, which in turn introduces additional forces on the distal stem as is illustrated in Fig. 5.33.

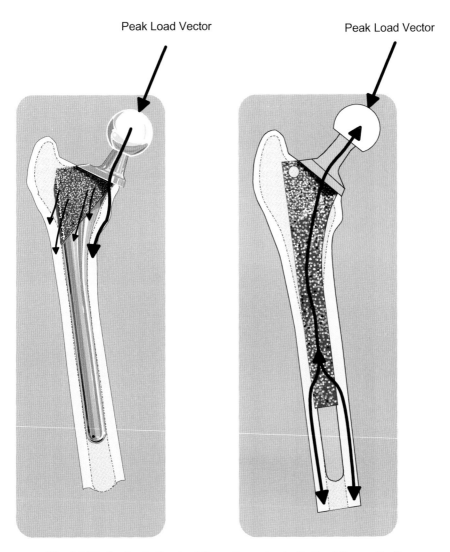

Fig. 5.34 Reduction in Proximal Stress Protection by Inclined Porous Coating.

d) Inclined Proximal Porous Coating

The initial B-P proximally coated, collared devices quickly developed resorption of the calcar under the collar as did other similar designs. Rather than eliminate the collar and use diaphyseal fixation it was decided to attempt to minimize such resorption with a collared device. Thus, in 1985 Buechel - Pappas introduced the use of a slanted proximal coating to prevent stress shielding of the calcar.

The absence of medial porous coating on the B-P Femoral Stem allows direct load transfer from the collar to the calcar producing more physiologic loading than collarless designs and designs which allow distal fixation. Thus, calcar stress protection is avoided.

The slanted coating configuration produces a load path that transfers load directly to the medial calcar region and distributes the load laterally, minimizing stress protection. Most coating configurations produce a load path that transfers the load distally bypassing the proximal femur, producing stress protection of the region.

Finite element analysis [101] and clinical experience [59] demonstrate that the distal slanted coating of the B-P Femoral Stem reduces stress protection and resorption of the proximal femur compared to fully, and one-third, coated stems. The gradual increase in coating length from the medial to lateral stem surfaces provides a gradual load transfer from prosthesis, to cancellous bone, and then to cortical bone, producing a gradual transfer of load to the lateral, distal cortex as shown in Fig. 5.34.

e) Proportional Sizing

Proportional proximal sizing in 1mm increments provides a close proximal fit and maximum proximal flare for torsional resistance to load. Torsional resistance is provided by the oval cross-section of this proximal flare and by the collar.

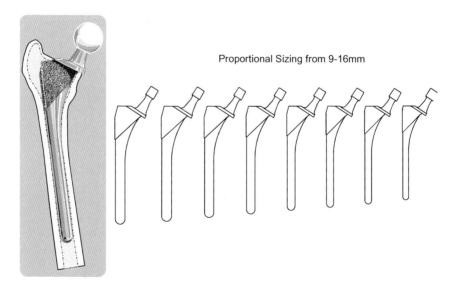

Proportional Sizing from 9-16mm

Fig. 5.35 Proportional Femoral Stem Sizing.

Finite element analysis demonstrates the important role the collar plays in resisting torsional loads [101]. Thus, torsion loads are transferred proximally, thereby avoiding torsional stress protection of the more distal regions and thus, transferring load more naturally than stems which resist torsional loads in the shaft. Such distal torsional restriction may contribute to the high incidence of thigh pain associated with designs that transfer load distally [59]. Clinical experience with the B-P Femoral Stem indicates a relatively low incidence of thigh pain [58, 59] which may be attributed to the lack of distal load transfer.

f) Ease of Removal

The use of lateral slots in the collar of the B-P Femoral Stem provides access to the anterior and posterior porous coating interfaces allowing resection of the interfaces in these regions if removal of the stem is required.

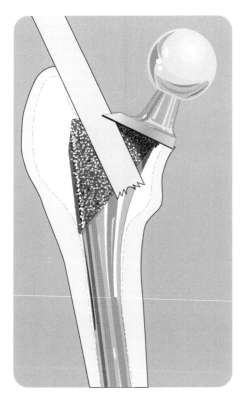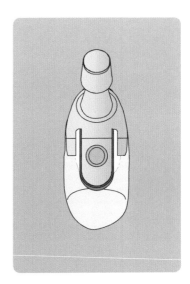

Fig. 5.36 Use of Calcar Collar Slots.

Now since the lateral porous coating interface is always accessible, and since there is little medial coating, the femoral component can be removed with little bone loss. A threaded removal hole is provided in the superior aspect of the stem allowing insertion of an impact-type removal instrument.

g)   Titanium Alloy and Ceramic TiN Coating

The greater flexibility of titanium alloy allows a greater share of the load to be carried by the bone than by the stiffer Co-Cr alloy. Thus, titanium alloy provides superior mechanical compatibility by reducing stress protection of bone. Further, titanium alloy is more biocompatible than Co-Cr alloy whose major components can be carcinogenic [123]. Finally, titanium alloy is stronger than Co-Cr alloy in both fatigue and yielding resistance [124]. Thus, except for the inferior abrasion resistance of titanium alloy, it is superior to Co-Cr alloys for use in implants.

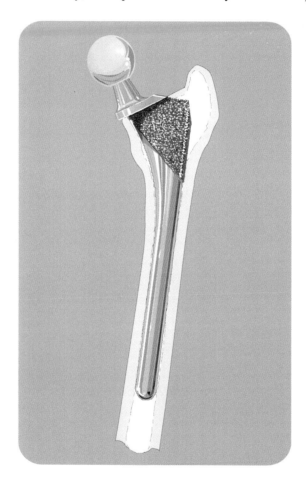

Fig. 5.37 TiN Ceramic Coated Titanium Alloy B-P Femoral Stem.

TiN ceramic finished stems provide enhanced biocompatibility. TiN is inert in vivo [125]. It shields the surface of the implant, particularly the porous coated region with its high surface area, against metallic ion release. The extreme hardness, and abrasion resistance, of TiN ceramic coatings has been shown to eliminate the metallosis observed in both uncoated titanium and Co-Cr alloy prostheses [126, 127]. This is because much less abrasion debris is generated, and the debris is inert and consists of nontoxic Ti and N ions. As a result, TiN ceramic finished titanium stems represent mechanically and biologically compatible femoral stems.

Retrieved specimens of femoral stems with modular heads have shown a disturbing degree of corrosion at the taper connection interface. This corrosion is the result of micro motion in the interface (fretting corrosion) and is present in both mixed and similar metal combinations [128].

Much of the micro motion in this interface is the result of excessive tolerances used in the manufacture of the tapers. The orthopaedic implant industry generally uses tolerances which are an order of magnitude greater than specified for normal machinery applications. To minimize this micro motion B-P Femoral Stems employ the same close tolerances used in the machinery industry.

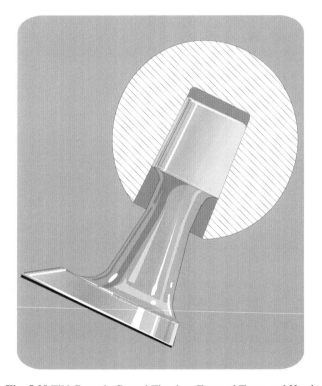

Fig. 5.38 TiN Ceramic Coated Titanium Femoral Taper and Head.

The use of TiN ceramic coating on the modular connection taper on the neck of the femoral stem, when used with a TiN ceramic finished titanium head, virtually eliminates corrosion at this interface since TiN ceramic coating and titanium are extremely resistant to fretting corrosion.

h)   Modular Femoral Stem and Stem Extensions

Modular Femoral Components are available in the same 8 sizes and have the same proximal configuration as the standard Femoral Component. These Modular Femoral Components are mated with a Stem Extension to produce a proper proximal and distal fit into the femur. Stem Extensions are available in a very large number of sizes. Lengths vary from 50 through 200mm in increments of 25mm. Diameters range from 9 through 20mm in 1mm increments. A modular Extended Collar Femoral Prosthesis is also available for revisions where there is significant proximal bone loss.

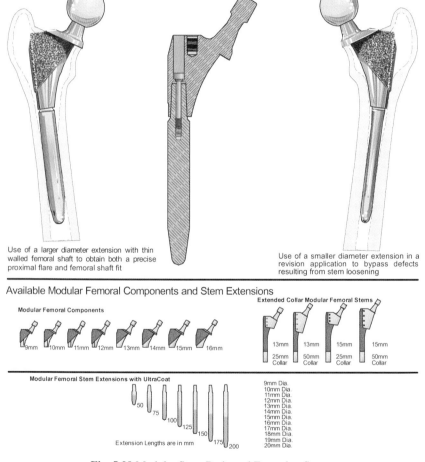

Fig. 5.39 Modular Stem Body and Extension System.

i) *Strength Analysis and Testing*

The basic assumption for the stem and extension strength calculations is that simple beam bending theory is adequate to predict the stresses. This assumption is conservative. The stem and extension can only see stresses resulting from bending, and much lower stresses resulting from possible axial stem tip loading. Ignoring this small compressive stress is conservative, since it tends to reduce the tensile stress component resulting from bending. It is this tensile stress which produces fatigue failure. The appropriate equations are found in Ref. [129] as are the stress concentration factors for the diameter transition regions of the internal stem tip and extension.

Using these equations and fatigue strengths of 240 MPa for Co-Cr and 400 MPa for Ti alloy (measured values after sintering and appropriate heat treatment) one finds the smallest (9mm) Buechel - Pappas (B-P) Modular Stem at its critical section is about as strong as a solid 12mm Co-Cr, one-third coated stem due to the greater strength of the Ti alloy. The B-P Modular Stem is about twice as strong as a 12mm fully, or five-eighths, porous coated Co-Cr stem due to the reduced strength resulting from stress concentrations from the sintered beads, and the fact that the substrate diameter of a 12 mm coated stem is only about 10.5mm.

Since titanium is much more flexible than Co-Cr, the bone into which the stem is implanted will carry more of the load. Thus, a Ti alloy stem will experience lower stresses than a Co-Cr stem [101]. Now, considering that modular B-P stems are equal in strength to, or stronger than, stems which have been in successful clinical use for an extended period of time without fracture, and that the loads carried by a Ti alloy stem are less than those carried by a Co-Cr stem, it is therefore, shown that the Ti alloy B-P Modular Stem is safe against fracture.

Consider now the extension. Using a conservative fatigue strength value of 524 MPa for wrought titanium alloy, the extension at its critical section is found to be stronger than the 12mm B-P stem. Thus, by the reasoning above the extension is also shown to be safe.

To evaluate experimentally the function of the extension connection six samples of the smallest Modular B-P Modular stems (9mm) with extensions were tested in a specially designed testing fixture. The mounts holding the specimens simulate the bending and extension properties of the human femur. The mounts are held and loaded in the fixture so as to simulate normal loading conditions during walking. The test was run in saline at a frequency of 4.8 Hz for 10 million cycles [130] as shown in Fig. 5.40.

Examination of the samples after testing found that there was no evidence of any damage, cracking, or deformation of the components. No wear or corrosion on the component interfaces was seen.

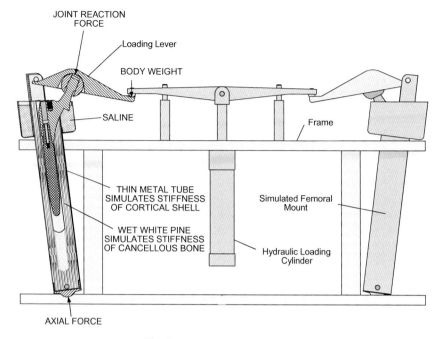

Fig. 5.40 Hip Loading Simulator.

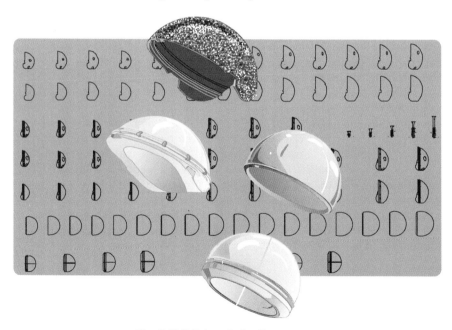

Fig. 5.41 B-P Acetabular Components.

5.4.3.2 The Acetabular Components

The B-P Total Hip Replacement System, as in most other current systems, has a large number of acetabular components to allow a broad range of patient sizes and pathologies. There are two types of cups, Fixed and Bipolar as shown in Fig. 5.41.

a) Fixed Cup
The fixed acetabular component uses a sintered bead, porous coated Titanium alloy outer shell of a partial hemispherical configuration and a "snap in" UHMWPe bearing. The system contains fixed component metal cups without screw holes, as well as five hole cups ranging from 45mm through 60mm in diameter, in 2mm increments as well as 6mm titanium screws in various lengths. The screws and cups with screw holes are intended for revision, or other cases, with sufficient acetabular erosion to require screw augmentation for stable fixation.

The anatomical cup configuration approximates the shape of the acetabulum and is recessed within its bony borders to minimize impingement and maximize range of motion. The spherical interface surface requires minimal bone resection and provides ease of acetabular preparation and intraoperative position adjustment.

Initially the bearing had only three locking tabs as illustrated in Fig. 5.42. Two disassociations of the bearing from the cup forced the use of additional tabs. No disassociations were noted after this change.

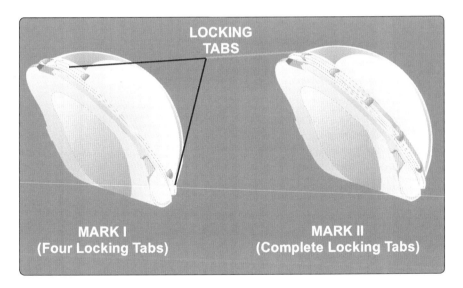

Fig. 5.42 Differences of the Mark I and Mark II bearing design locking mechanisms.

Bearings are available to fit these cups with internal diameters that fit 22, 28, and 32mm femoral heads.

1) Anatomical Configuration

The fixed acetabular cup and bearing insert are configured to approximate the shape of the natural acetabulum. The outside edges of both the fixed cup and bearing insert are recessed within the bony borders of the acetabulum.

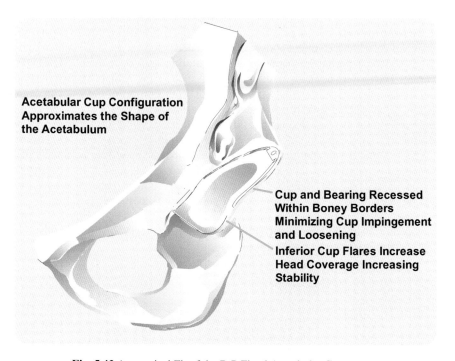

Acetabular Cup Configuration Approximates the Shape of the Acetabulum

Cup and Bearing Recessed Within Boney Borders Minimizing Cup Impingement and Loosening

Inferior Cup Flares Increase Head Coverage Increasing Stability

Fig. 5.43 Anatomical Fit of the B-P Fixed Acetabular Components.

2) Recessed Positioning

Recessing the fixed cup and bearing insert within the bony borders of the acetabulum minimizes potential impingement of the components with the femur or femoral components. This reduces the potential for impingement torque which can contribute to fixed cup loosening or bearing insert separation. Further, avoidance of impingement from protruding acetabular components maximizes the range of motion of the hip, reducing the potential for subluxation resulting from such impingement as shown in Fig. 5.44.

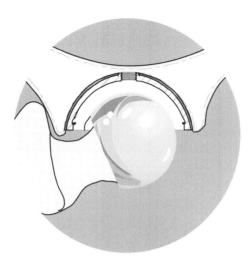

Fig. 5. 44 Recessed Acetabular Cup Avoids Neck Impingement.

3)   *Spherical Fixation Surface*

The spherical shape of the acetabular cup requires minimal removal of bone during acetabular preparation using ordinary acetabular reamers. The angular orientation of the cup is not dependent on the preparation procedure and may be adjusted for optimal position.

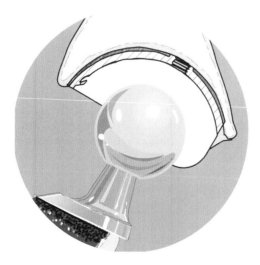

Fig. 5.45 Spherical Fixation Surface.

4)   *Improved Dislocation Resistance*

Mimicking the natural acetabulum, the fixed acetabular component has anterior and posterior flares which increase the inferior engagement between the femoral head and the acetabular bearing producing enhanced joint stability, particularly during flexion.

5)   *Fixed Cup Position*

The fixed acetabular cup is designed to be implanted with its face at 30° from the horizontal and in 20° of anteversion.

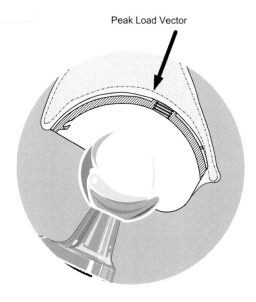

Fig. 5.46 Alignment of the B-P Fixed Acetabular Component with the Peak Load Vector.

At this orientation, it is aligned with the Peak Load Vector resulting from normal walking activity [3]. Such alignment produces greater uniformity of compressive stress at the prosthesis – to - bone interface providing more favorable conditions for establishing and maintaining fixation. In particular, undesirable tensile stresses at this interface resulting from tipping loads are minimized by such alignment. Further, alignment of the cup with peak load vector and, thus, the neck axis optimizes range of motion as well as interface loading conditions.

6)   *Enhanced Biocompatibility*

Titanium alloy is used for the Fixed Acetabular Cup since it is more biocompatible than Co-Cr alloy whose major components can be carcinogenic [123]. Biocompatibility can be further enhanced by the application of ceramic coating on titanium. TiN ceramic is inert in vivo [127]. It shields the surface of the implant, particularly the porous coated region with its high surface area, against metallic ion release. As a result, titanium acetabular cups with ceramic coating represent the most biologically compatible metallic cups available.

b) Bipolar Cup
Experience [66-72] with these devices and analysis of their design and behavior has provided criteria for their evaluation and selection. On the basis of this experience one can conclude that the selection of a multicomponent proximal femoral endoprosthesis involves a consideration of:

1) Positioning
Some devices [31] utilize negative eccentricity between the centers of the internal (femoral component head to bearing insert) and external metal cup to acetabulum articulation so that the external articulation center falls proximally relative to the internal center as shown in Fig. 5.47.

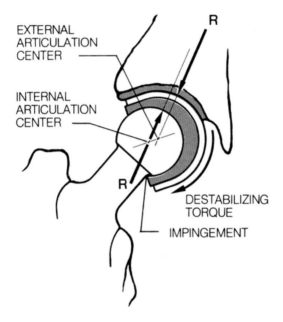

Fig. 5.47 Negative Eccentricity.

Such a configuration produces a destabilizing torque which holds the cup in extreme varus. This reduces internal articulation by virtue of enforced internal prosthetic impingement and provides an undesirable load bearing configuration.

Devices with neutral eccentricity [29] partially avoid this problem but fail to exploit the potential benefits of positive eccentricity used in some of the newest generation cups. Neutral eccentricity devices are typified by a highly variable positioning of the acetabular component. Positive eccentricity [32], such as used in the Self Centering Universal Hip, can be used to provide more consistently desirable acetabular component cup position. Here (as shown in Fig. 5.48) the eccentricity produces a stabilizing torque tending to align the acetabular component axis with the joint reaction force. This provides an excellent load bearing configuration, maximizes head to bearing motion and minimizes internal prosthetic impingement.

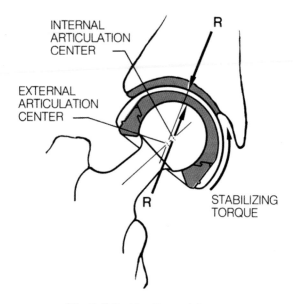

Fig. 5.48 Positive Eccentricity.

2) Wear
A study of MIT and the Harvard Medical School show the linear wear rate of the 22 mm head to be 100% higher than the 32 mm size [65]. Thus, the larger head reduces geometric changes which tend to inhibit the internal prosthetic range of motion. A study by Gold and Walker [131] shows the volumetric wear rate for a 22 mm head against ultra high molecular weight polyethylene (UHMWPE) to be about 60% higher than for a 32 mm head. Such reduction in wear debris by use of a 32 mm head would substantially reduce any adverse reaction to polyethylene wear particles [131, 132].

3) Internal Range of Motion
A primary object of the multicomponent (bipolar) femoral endoprosthesis is to conserve acetabular stock by substituting internal prosthetic articulation for external acetabular articulation. Thus, a large internal articulation range of motion should be desirable for such prostheses. Unfortunately, a large or increased range of internal motion in acetabular components employing negative or neutral eccentricity can result in an increase in varus positioning or variation in positioning respectively and therefore a large range of motion is undesirable in such devices. Thus, some prostheses have a relatively small range of motion so as to place limits on positioning extremes.

   Use of positive eccentricity however assures proper acetabular component
positioning. Thus such designs can fully exploit the benefits of a large internal
articulation range. Such devices must, however, have a sufficiently large range of
motion to avoid impingement between the neck of the femoral stem and the
acetabular component as the result of the enforced valgus orientation resulting
from the stabilizing couple.

4)   Ease of Reduction

Although post-operative dislocation as shown in Figs. 5.49 and 5.50 is not a
frequent occurrence, it occurs frequently enough [70-72] so that design features
affecting the ability to reduce the prosthesis should be considered in selection. On
dislocation, the cup face with edge distance "A" may be caught on the acetabular
rim or associated soft tissue preventing closed reduction. Open reduction may also
become necessary as the result of component separation after joint dislocation or
during an attempt at closed reduction after such dislocation.

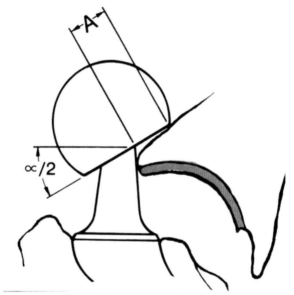

Fig. 5.49 Dislocation and Impingement.

This situation is illustrated in Fig. 5.50.

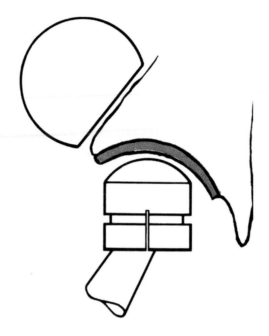

Fig. 5.50 Component Separation.

A reduction in edge distance "A" and an increase in the face angle of α/2 (α is the internal range of motion) make such a situation less likely and increase prospects for closed reduction. Reduction may be further aided by use of a beveled face as shown in Fig. 5.51.

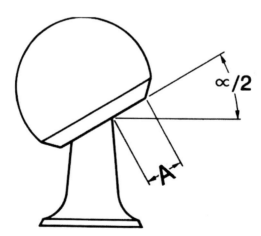

Fig. 5.51 Use of bevel to reduce edge distance.

Use of a 32 mm head further reduces the "A" dimension providing still more favorable conditions for reduction as shown in Fig. 5.52.

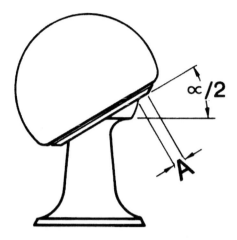

Fig. 5.52 Use of 32 mm head to reduce edge distance.

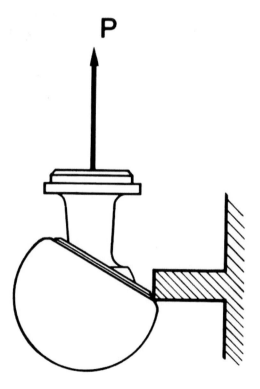

Fig. 5.53 Component Separation Force Test.

The separation strength of the assembly should also be considered since even with use of a favorable face configuration, considerable separation forces may be encountered after dislocation. This strength can be estimated with reasonable accuracy by use of the separation force test as illustrated in Fig. 5.53.

5) System Flexibility

A major advantage of the multicomponent system is that available acetabular components and stems can be combined to produce a large variety of configurations thus allowing a close match between availability and requirement. For example, use of 10 acetabular components sizes with 10 different stems, a practical offering of components, can produce 100 variations. Such a large number of variations would be impractical to offer in a single component system. Thus, the multicomponent system offers greater flexibility of application.

6) Ease of Assembly and Disassembly

Intra-operative considerations such as ease of prosthetic component assembly and disassembly and the nature of the instrumentation are also important in system selection. Only the "Self Centering" and "UHR" systems allow assembly with minimal digital pressure without use of special instruments. These systems also allow easy disassembly by use of simple release instruments.

7) Comparison

Table 5.6 summarizes the properties of various multicomponent femoral head replacement systems. From this data the orthopaedic surgeon can readily apply the considerations presented here to select the best system for his patients. Reviewing this table it may be seen that most designs apparently have serious design deficiencies.

Table 5.6 Comparison of Several Multicomponent Endoprosthesis.

*Values given are for 48 mm or 49 mm metal cup and 32 mm femoral head where available.

PROSTHESIS SYSTEM DESIGNATION	Eccentricity	α Degrees	32 mm Head Option	Edge Distance A. mm	Face Angle α/2. Degrees	Beveled Face	Separation Force Newton (lbs.)	Acetabular Component Dia. Available mm	Femoral Head Sizes, mm	Adaptability, mm Stem Choice	Special Femoral Trials Needed	Separate Bearing Insert	Assembly with minimal digital pressure	Disassembly with minimal force and simple instrument
SELF-CENTERING (De Puy)	Pos.	71	Yes	5	35½	Yes	2180 (490)	39-57	32 & 22	great	No	Yes	Yes	Yes
UPF (3 M)	Neu.	55	No	20	27½	No	40 (9)	41-60	22	limited	Yes	Yes	No	Yes
UHR (Osteonics)	Pos.	50	No	17	25	Yes	396 (89)	41-61	22	limited	Yes	No	Yes	Yes
GILBERTY (Zimmer)	Neg.	90	Yes	14	45	No	67 (15)	42-57	32	great	No	No	No	No
BI-CENTRIC (Howmedica)	Neg.	84	Yes	13	42	No	151 (34)	41-55	32, 26, & 22	great	No	No	No	No

The UPF, Gilberty & Bi-Centric [133] devices appear to have insufficient resistance against separation. The UHR [134] has a range of motion apparently insufficient to prevent serious impingement between the acetabular component and the femoral component neck. Furthermore, the relatively large range of motion of the Gilberty and Bi-Centric prostheses only increases the problems associated with the negative eccentricity of these devices. Thus the surgeon must exercise due caution in his evaluation and selection of a Bipolar hip replacement prosthesis.

8)   *Reduced Acetabular Erosion and Metallic Debris*
The B-P hip system employs TiN ceramic on its Universal Self-Aligning Acetabular Metal Component because its smoothness, and resulting low friction, should reduce erosion of the articular cartilage. Further, its hardness and biocompatibility should minimize the release of potentially harmful metallic debris which may result from the metal cup to acetabular articulation.

5.4.3.3   Total Hip Replacement Range of Motion

Computer solid models provide a convenient tool for the study of prosthetic range of motion and stability. Current designs show considerable variation in range of motion and stability. Relatively simple and economical computer methods can be used to evaluate the ROM and stability of existing hip designs. These methods are useful in the development of improved designs.

Computer solid models of the acetabular component and the head, neck, and collar of the femoral component of B-P designs where generated using the Autodesk AME solid modeling package on a PC. The center of the femoral head was placed coincident with the center of the spherical surface of the acetabular bearing. The stem was rotated about axis through the femoral head until impingement was observed. The stability at the point of impingement was then evaluated from the amount of engagement of the femoral head and acetabular bearing. The axes used are those associated with; flexion - extension, internal - external rotation, ab-adduction. Additionally combinations of these motions were studied in order to develop a motion envelope for the devices tested.

The larger 32mm femoral head designs generally provided motion and stability superior to smaller diameter heads.

Table 5.7 Neck-Socket Contact Angles of Prosthetic Components B-P Total Hip Replacement System.

	28mm Head, STD. Neck	32mm Head, STD. Neck
Anteversion (Fem. /Acet.)	10/20	10/20
Inclination (Fem. /Acet.)	25/30	25/30
Flexion	100	102
Extension	62	63
Abduction	79	79
Adduction	56	66
Internal Rotation	185	213
External Rotation	120	148

Note: All numbers are in degrees. Measured at neutral position.

Comparing this data to normal motion given in Section 5.2.1 it may be seen that the B-P total Hip provides an ample ROM except in flexion. Dislocations as the result of hyperflexion have been observed with this design, probably the result of lower than normal flexion available with this device. Patients should, therefore, be advised to limit full flexion to about 100°.

5.4.3.4 The Resurfacing Total Hip Replacement

The B-P carefully designed, thin wall, Resurfacing Femoral Cup requires minimal femoral bone removal and allows use of an acetabular cup which requires minimal reaming of the acetabular cavity. Size selection is therefore based on the requirement for acetabular resurfacing rather than femoral resurfacing. Thus, hip resurfacing is now truly conservative as it avoids over reaming of the socket.

TiN ceramic coating on the Femoral Component should reduce bearing wear and friction below that of cobalt-chromium femoral heads used in conventional stem type prostheses [58].

A non-porous coated, smooth, straight tapered stem is used to align the Femoral Cup during impaction and mechanically wedges the prosthesis into place for immediate stability. This configuration minimizes compressive stem load transfer to the shaft while providing protection against shearing of the femoral neck.

In addition, the Acetabular Fixation Cup accepts both the B-P hip system's 32 and 28mm Acetabular Bearings allowing revision to femoral stem prosthesis in the event of resorption under the Femoral Component or fracture of the femoral neck, without removing a well fixed acetabular cup.

5.4.4 Remaining Problems

5.4.4.1 Cysts

Wear particle disease in the form of osteolysis of bone has become a significant problem after "resurfacing" total hip replacement, just as in "stem-type" total hip replacement. Fine polyethylene (UHMWPe) particles, often in the submicron range have been identified in cysts found in the femoral head and neck; the ilium, ischium and pubic ramus. These "osteolytic cysts" begin to develop 3 to 4 years after surgery in a high percentage of patients who are sensitized to these particles. They are usually painless and imperceptible to the patient and are only discovered by routine x-ray evaluation during the yearly follow-up examinations.

If progression of cystic size is seen over a one to two year interval, a CT scan of the hip and pelvis is recommended to evaluate the location, volume and extent of the cysts. If they become expansile, a femoral neck fracture or acetabular cup migration can occur, causing significant pain and failure of the hip replacement.

Treatment is directed at curettage and bone grafting of all cystic lesions greater than 1 cm. and replacing the polyethylene with a more durable and wear resistant bearing. In some cases, when the femoral neck has significantly resorbed ("penciled") or fractured, a femoral stem-type revision is necessary to restore proper femoral loading mechanics.

When massive osteolysis of the pelvis is associated with migration of the acetabular cup, extensive bone grafting accompanied by pelvic augmentation with a "cage" or "jumbo cup" may be necessary to recreate a stable and properly oriented acetabular cup that provides proper loading and resists dislocation.

5.4.4.2 Wear

The greatest challenge to long-term survival of hip joint replacement is the ability to resist wear. Wear is equally as important as fixation and anatomic motion in terms of reproducing an idealized joint replacement reconstruction. Fixation and motion in the hip have been consistently reproduced over the past 30 years, but wear has been variable despite the use of various "bearing couples", namely, metal-polyethylene, ceramic-polyethylene, ceramic-ceramic and metal-metal. Each bearing material has had its own peculiar problems.

Metal-metal bearings are associated with persistent ten-fold elevations of metal ions [56] that have been associated with chromosomal abnormalities, [57] bringing into question their long-term use in younger patients for whom they were intended.

Ceramic-ceramic bearings have had excellent wear properties when components are properly aligned, without "neck-cup impingement" problems. Unfortunately, ceramic-ceramic bearings can develop a clinical "squeak" in up to 10% of cases [39, 135] causing patient apprehension in some devices. Still, properly designed and implanted ceramic-on-ceramic total hip devices can apparently provide twenty years of service due to their excellent biocompatible wear properties [33-37].

Metal-polyethylene has been used predominantly for total hip replacement over the past 40 years. This combination has provided dramatic "life-improvement" for millions of patients, but over time has been involved with "osteolytic cysts" after long-term use, a normal consequence of conventional polyethylene wear [35]. Enhanced polyethylenes, known as highly cross-linked, have been developed using an increased irradiation and annealing process to improve wear properties [136]. Clinical studies [137] have supported some hip simulator studies [138] in describing major improvements in wear properties over conventional polyethylene. These improvements may allow metal or ceramic-polyethylene bearings to last a lifetime for middle-aged or elderly patients undergoing this procedure.

5.4.5 The Future

Based on the performance of the fifth generation it seems doubtful that, except for a possible increase in the ROM in flexion, further design refinement can achieve significant performance improvement with the availability of currently validated materials. Such improvement must come from material improvements or the development of new materials.

5.5 Conclusion

Charnley opened the door to successful hip arthroplasty in the late 1950's. His third generation hip arthroplasty device is still used today in essentially the same form as it had in the 1960's.

The fourth generation yielded some conceptual improvements, but not apparently in long term use. Even in the short term fourth generation, biologically fixed devices such as the AML had significant problems such as thigh pain which are much less prevalent in cemented, third generation designs.

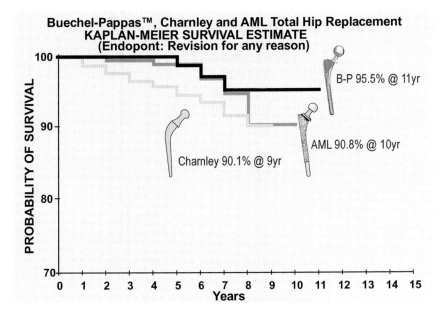

Fig. 5.54 Comparison of survival of Typical Third, Fourth and Fifth Generation Total Hip Arthroplasties.

Knowledge about these earlier designs, technical advances and careful analysis of their performance allowed the development of a fifth generation. This effort produced improved performance of hip systems making them comparable to most total knee replacements as shown by the survival analysis in Fig. 5.54.

Still the longevity of the fifth generation design is inferior to the better mobile bearing knee designs. An improvement in the wear properties of the materials used must be made to attain the same performance as the best knee replacements [139]. Hopefully potential solutions, such as highly cross-linked UHMWPe or improved ceramics, will provide such improvement.

References

[1] Roach, K.E., Miles, T.P.: Normal Hip and Knee Active Range of Motion: The relationship to Age. Physical Therapy 71, 657 (1991)

[2] Lea, R.D., Gerhardt, J.J.: Range-of Motion Measurements. JBJS(Am) 77, 784 (1995)

[3] Paul, J.P.: Load Actions on the Human Femur in Walking and Some Resultant Stresses. Experimental Mechanics 11(3), 121–127 (1971)

[4] Crowninshield, R.D., et al.: A Biomechanical Investigation of the Human Hip. J. Biomech. 11, 75 (1978)

[5] Rydell, N.W.: Forces Acting on the Femoral Head Prosthesis: A Study on Strain Gauge Supplied Prosthesis in Living Persons. Acta Orthop. Scand. 88(supp.) (1966)

[6] Davy, D.T., et al.: Telemetric Force Measurements across the Hip after Total Arthroplasty. JBJS 70A, 45 (1988)

[7] Johnston, R.C., Brand, R.A.: Reconstruction of the hip - A Mathematical Approach to Determine Optimum Geometric Relationships. JBJS 61A, 639 (1979)

[8] Peters, C.L., Erickson, J.A.: Treatment of femoro-acetabular impingement with surgical dislocation and debridement in young adults. J. Bone Joint Surg. Am. 88(8), 1735–1741 (2006)

[9] Standaert, C.J., Manner, P.A., Herring, S.A.: Expert opinion and controversies in musculoskeletal and sports medicine: Femoroacetabular impingement. Arch. Phys. Med. Rehabil. 89(5), 890–893 (2008)

[10] Philippon, M.J., Briggs, K.K., Yen, Y.M., Kuppersmith, D.A.: Outcomes following hip arthroscopy for femoroacetabular impingement with associated chondrolabral dysfunction: Minimum two-year follow-up. J. Bone Joint Surg. Br. 91(1), 16–23 (2009)

[11] Bardakos, N.V., Villar, R.N.: Predictors of progression of osteoarthritis in femoroacetabular impingement: A radiological study with a minimum of ten years follow-up. J. Bone Joint Surg. Br. 91(2), 162–169 (2009)

[12] Beaulè, P.E., Allen, D.J., Clohisy, J.C., et al.: The young adult with hip impingement: Deciding on the optimal intervention. J. Bone Joint Surg. Am. 91(1), 210–221 (2009)

[13] Amstutz, H.C., Clark, I.C.: Evolution of Hip Arthroplasty. In: He, A. (ed.) Hip Arthroplasty, Ch. I. Churchill Livingstone, New York (1991)

[14] Smith-Petersen, M.N.: Arthroplasty of the Hip: A New Method. JBJS 21, 269 (1939)

[15] Gluck, T.H.: Arch. Klin. Chir., vol. 41, p. 234 (1891)

[16] Wiles, P.: The Surgery of the Osteoarthritic Hip. Br. J. Surg. 45, 488 (1958)

[17] Smith-Petersen, M.N.: Evolution of Mold Arthroplasty of the Hip Joint. JBJS 30B, 59 (1948)

[18] Urist, M.: The Principles of Hip-Socket Arthroplasty. JBJS 39A, 786 (1957)

[19] McBride, E.D.: The Flanged Acetabular Replacement Prosthesis. Arch. Surg. 83, 786 (1961)

[20] Judet, J., Judet, R.: The Use of an Artificial Femoral Head for Arthroplasty of the Hip Joint. JBJS(Br) 32, 166 (1950)

[21] Heywood, M.B.: Use of the Austin Moore Prosthesis for Advanced Osteoarthritis of the Hip. JBJS(Br) 48, 236 (1966)

[22] Browett, J.B.: The Uncemented Thompson Prosthesis. JBJS(Br) 63, 635 (1981)

[23] McKee, E.D., Watson-Farrar, J.: Replacement of arthritic Hips by the McKee-Farrar Prosthesis. JBJS (Br) 48, 245 (1966)

[24] Charnley, J.: Low Friction Arthroplasty of the Hip. Springer, New York (1979)

[25] Charnley, J., et al.: The Optimum Size of Prosthetic Heads in Relation to Wear of Plastic Sockets in Total Replacement of the Hip. Medical Biological Engineering 7, 31 (1969)

[26] Muller, M.E.: Total Hip Prosthesis. Clin. Ortho. 72, 46 (1970)

[27] Catalog, D.: Section A, DePuy, Warsaw IN (1983)

[28] Ring, P.A.: Complete Replacement Arthroplasty of the Hip by the Ring Prosthesis. JBJS (BR) 50, 720 (1968)

[29] Bateman, J.E.: Single Assembly Total Hip Prosthesis - Preliminary Report. Orthop. Digest. 2, 15 (1944)

[30] Christensen, T.: A Combined Endo and Total Prosthesis with Trunion Bearing. Acta Chir. Scand. 140, 185 (1974)

[31] Gilberty, R.: A New Concept of Bipolar Endoprosthesis. Orthop. Rev. 3, 40 (1974)

[32] Pappas, M.J., et al.: Eccentricity in Universal Type Proximal Femoral Endoprostheses: Biomechanical and Clinical Analysis. In: Transactions of the Eighth Annual Meeting of the Society for Biomaterials, vol. V (1982)

[33] Boutin, P.: Total arthroplasty of the hip by fritted aluminum prostheses - Experimental study and 1st clinical applications. Rev. Chir. Orthop. Reparatrice Appar. Mot. 58, 229–246 (1972) (French)

[34] Mamadouche, M., et al.: Alumina-on alumina Total Hip Arthroplasty - A Minimum 18. 5- Year5 Follow-ip Study. JBJS 84A(1), 69–77 (2002)

[35] Granchi, D., et al.: Immuniligical changes in patients with primary osteoarthritis of the hip after total joint replacement. JBJS 85B(5), 758–764 (2003)

[36] Bierbaum, B.E., et al.: Ceramic-on-Ceramic Bearing in Total Hip Arthroplasty. Clin. Orthop. Relat. Res. 405, 158–163 (2002)

[37] Nizard, R., et al.: Alumina-on-Alumina Hip Arthroplasty in Patients Younger Than 30 Years Old. Clin. Orthop. Relat. Res. 466, 317–323 (2008)

[38] Toni, A., et al.: Fracture of ceramic components in total hip arthroplasty, 1120-7000/049-08$04.00/0 (2009)

[39] Keurentjes, J.V., et al.: High Incidence of Squeaking in THAs with Alumina Ceramic-on-ceramic Bearings. Clin. Orthop. Relat. Res. 446, 1438–1443 (2008)

[40] Gerard, Y., et al.: Hip Arthroplasty by Matching Cups. Rev. Clin. Orthop. 60(supplement 2), 281 (1974)

[41] Amstutz, H.C., et al.: A Total Hip Replacement by Eccentric Shells. Clin. Orthop. 128, 261 (1977)

[42] Furuya, K., et al.: Socket Cup Arthroplasty. Clin. Orthop. 134, 41 (1978)

[43] Freeman, M.A.R., et al.: Cemented Double Cup Arthroplasty of the Hip: A five Year Experience with the ICLH Prosthesis. Clin. Ortho. 134, 46 (1978)

[44] Wagner, H.: Surface Replacement Arthroplasty of the Hip. Clin. Orthop. 134, 102 (1978)

[45] Judet, et al.: A Noncemented Total Hip Prosthesis. Clin. Orthop. 137(76) (1978)

[46] Lord, G.A., et al.: An Uncemented Total Hip Prosthesis. Clin. Orthop. 141, 2 (1979)

[47] Pilliar, R.M.: Porous Surfaced Layered Prosthetic Devices. Biomed. Eng. 10, 126 (1975)

[48] Gelante, J., et al.: Sintered Fiber Metal Composite as a Basis for Attachment of Metal to Bone. JBJS 53A, 101 (1971)

[49] Noble, P.C., et al.: The Myth of 'Press-Fit' in the Proximal Femur. Baylor College of Medicine (1999)

[50] Engh, et al.: Biological Fixation of a Moore Prosthesis. Orthopedics 7, 28 (1984)

[51] Mittelmeir, H.: Zementlose Verankerung von Endoprosthes nach dem Tragrippenprinzip. Z. Ortop. 176, 53 (1974)

[52] Lord, G., Bancel, P.: An Uncemented Total Hip Replacement: Experimental Study and Review of 300 Madreporique Arthroplasties. Clin. Orthop. 141, 2 (1979)

[53] Harris, W.H., et al.: Socket Fixation using a metal backed Acetabular Cups for Total Hip Replacement. JBJS 64A, 745 (1982)

[54] Schmaizried, T.P., et al.: The Role of Acetabular Component Screw Holes and/or Screws in the Development of Pelvic Osteolysis. In: Proc. Inst. Mech. Eng., vol. 2(13), p. 147 (1999)

[55] Robinson, E., et al.: Minimum 7- Year Outcome of Birmingham Hip Resurfacing (BHP): A Review of 1354 Cases from an International Register. The Robert Jones & Agnes Hunt Orthopaedic & District Hospital NHS Trust, Oswestry Shropshire, UK (2008)

[56] Nevelos, J., et al.: Development, Validation and Multi-Centre Follow -up- of a Modern Metal-On-Metal Hip Resurfacing Prosthesis. In: AAOS Scientific Exhibit (2004)

[57] Dunston, E., et al.: Chromosomal Aberration in the Peripheral Blood of Patients with Metal-on-Metal Hip Bearings. JBJS 90A, 517–522 (2008)

[58] Buechel, F.F., et al.: Two to 12- Year Evaluation of Cementless Buechel-Pappas Total Hip Arthroplasty. J. of Arthroplasty 19(8), 1017–1027 (2004)

[59] Hamlin, F.D., Buechel, F.F., Pappas, M.J.: Stress Shielding As It Relates to Proximally Porous Coated Femoral Stems of Varying Configurations: A 10 Year Cementless Total Hip Replacement Study. Journal of Orthopaedic Rheumatology 6, 2–3 (1993)

[60] Coll, B.F., et al.: Surface Modification of Medical implants and Surgical Devices Using TiN Layers. Surface and Coating Technology 36 (1988)

[61] Pappas, M.J., Makris, G., Buechel, F.F.: Titanium Nitride Ceramic Film against polyethylene: A 48 Million Cycle Wear Test. Clinical Orthopaedics and Related Research 317 (1995)

[62] Pappas, M.J., Makris, G., Buechel, F.F.: Wear in Prosthetic Knee Joints. Presented at the 59th Annual Meeting of The American Academy of Orthopaedic Surgeons Scientific Exhibit., Washington, DC (1992)

[63] Pappas, M.J., et al.: Comparison of Wear of UHMWPe Cups Articulating with Co-Cr and TiN Coated Femoral Heads. Transactions of the Society of Biomaterials III (1990)

[64] Freeman, M.A.R., Bobyn, D., Buechel, F.F.: Evolving Technologies: Old Problems and New Answers. Presented at the Ninth Annual Current Concepts in Joint Replacement, Orlando, Florida(Panel Discussion) (1993)

[65] Weightman, B., Paul, I.L., Rose, R., Rodin, E.L.: A Comparative Study of Total Hip Replacement Prostheses. Journal of Biomechanics 6, 299–312 (1973)

[66] Drinker, H., Murray, W.R.: The Universal Proximal Femoral Endoprosthesis: Short-Term Comparison with Conventional Hemiarthroplasty. JBJS 61A(8), 1167–1174 (1979)

[67] Goldie, I.F., Raner, C.: Total Hip Replacement with a Trunion Bearing Prosthesis: Biomechanical Principles and Preliminary Clinical Results. Acta Orthop. Scand. 50, 205–216 (1979)

[68] Langan, P., Weiss, G.A.: Stability of the Gilberty Bipolar Hip: Report of Three Cases. Clinical Orthop. & Related Res. 137, 129–131 (1978)

[69] Long, W.J., Knight, W.: Bateman VPF Prosthesis in Fractures of the Femoral Neck. Clinical Orthop. and Related Res. 152, 198–201 (1980)

[70] Anderson, P.R., Milgram, J.W.: Dislocation and Component Separation of the Bateman Hip Endoprosthesis. JAMA 240(19), 2079–2080 (1978)

[71] Barmada, R., Siege, I.M.: Postoperative Separation of the Femoral and Acetabular Components of a Single- Assembly Total Hip (Bateman) Replacement: Report of Two Cases. JBJS 61A(5), 777–779 (1979)

[72] Ahlgren, D., Lemperg, R.: Dislocation of a Total Hip Prosthesis of the Christiansen Type: A Case Report. Acta Orthop. Scanda. 45, 742–745 (1974)

[73] Yamanoto, T., et al.: Wear analysis of retrieved ceramic-on ce3ramic articulations in total hip arthroplasty: Femoral head makes contact with the rim of the socket outside the bearing surface. J. Biomed. Mat. Res. 73B(2), 301–307 (2005)

[74] Mai, K., et al.: Early Dislocation Rate in Ceramic-on-Ceramic Total Hip Arthroplasty. HSS J. 4, 10–13 (2008)

[75] Walker, W.L., Yeung, E.: A Review of Squeaking Hips. J. Am. Acad. Orthop. Surg. 18(6), 319–326 (2010)

[76] Restrepo, C., et al.: The Effect of Stem Design on the Prevalence of Squeaking Following Ceramic-on-Ceramic Bearing Total Hip Arthroplasty. JBJS 92A, 550–557 (2010)

[77] D' Antonio, J., et al.: Alumina Ceramic Bearings for Total Hip Arthroplasty: Five-year Results of a Prospective Randomized Study. Clin. Orthop. Relat. Res. 436, 164–171 (2005)

[78] Savarino, L., et al.: Is wear debris responsible for failure in alumina-on-alumina implants? Acta Orthopaedica 80(2), 162–167 (2009)

[79] Engh, C.A., Zettl-Schaffer, K.F., Kukita, Y., et al.: Histological and Radiographic Assessment of Well Functioning Porous-Coated Acetabular Components. JBJS 75A, 814–824 (1993)

[80] Engh, C.A., Bobyn, D.B.: The influence of stem size and extent of porous coating on femoral bone resorption after primary cementless hip arthroplasty. Clin. Orthop. 231, 7–28 (1988)

[81] Engh, C.A., Massin, P., Sutters, K.E.: Roentgenographic Assessment of the biologic fixation of porous-surfaced femoral components. Clin. Orthop. 257, 107–128 (1990)

[82] Burkart, B.C., Bourne, R.B., Rorabeck, C.H., et al.: Thigh Pain in Cementless Total Hip Arthroplasty: A Comparison of Two Systems at 2-Year Follow-Up. Orthop. Clinic of NA 24, 645–653 (1993)

[83] Haddad, R.J., et al.: A Comparison of Three Varieties of Non-Cemented Porous Coated Hip Replacement. JBJS 75B (1990)

[84] Engh, C.A., Massin, P.: Cementless total hip arthroplasty using the anatomic medullary locking stem. Clin. Orthop. 249, 141–158 (1989)

[85] Engh, C.A., Bobyn, J.D., Glassmann, A.H.: Porous coated hip replacement. The factors governing bone ingrowth, stress shielding and clinical results. JBJS 69B, 45–55 (1987)

[86] Schmalzreid, T.P., Jasty, M., Harris, W.H.: The Harris-Galante porous-coated acetabular component with screw fixation. JBJS 74A, 1130–1139 (1992)

[87] Martin, J.W., Branam, L., Whiteside, L.: Comparison of the Rate of Osteolysis in Two Types of Porous Coated Cementless Tibial Components. Presented at the 61st Annual American Academy of Orthopaedic Surgeons Meeting, New Orleans, Louisiana (Scientific Exhibit) (1994)

[88] Harris, W.: The Problem: Osteolysis. Presented at the 22nd Open Scientific Meeting of The Hip Society, New Orleans, Louisiana (1994)

[89] Engh Jr., C.A., et al.: Long-Term Results of Use of the Anatomic Medullary Locking Prosthesis in total Hip Arthroplasty. JBJS 79A, 177 (1995)

[90] Engh, et al.: Long Term Result using the Anatomic Medullary Locking Hip Prosthesis. Clin. Orthop. 393, 137 (2001)

[91] Dawson, J., Jameson-Shorthall, E., Emeron, M., et al.: Issues relating to Long-Term Follow-up in Hip Arthroplasty Surgery: A review of 598 cases at 7 years comparing 2 prostheses using revision rates, survival analysis and Patient-based measures. Journ. of Arthop. 15, 710–717 (2000)

[92] Herberts, P., Malchau, H., Romanus, B.: Uncemented Total Hip Replacements in young Adults. In: Scientific Exhibit 55th Annual Meeting AAOS at Atlanta, Georgia (1988)

[93] Greenwald, A.S., Froimson, A.I., Postak, P.O., et al.: Cup/Liner Incongruity of Two Piece Acetabular Designs: A Factor in Clinical Failure. Presented at the 61st Annual American Academy of Orthopaedic Surgeons Meeting at New Orleans, Louisiana (Scientific Exhibit) (1994)

[94] Dorr, L.D.: Fixation of the acetabular component: the case for cementless bone ingrowth modular sockets. Arthroplasty 11(1), 3–6 (1996)

[95] Buechel, F.F.: A practical modification of The Harris Hip Scoring Scale for use by Orthopaedic Residents. N.J Orthopaedic Hospital Reprint (1978)

[96] DeLee, J.G., Charnley, J.: Radiological Demarcation of Cemented Sockets in Total Hip Replacement. Clin. Orthop. 121, 20–32 (1978)

[97] Drucker, D., Buechel, F.F., Pappas, M.J.: Evolution of the Porous-Coated Hemispherical. Acetabular Cup For Application in Total Hip Replacement: An Eight Year Clinical Study (unpublished)

[98] Gruen, T.A., McNiece, G.M., Amstutz, H.C.: Modes of failure of cemented stem type femoral components: A Radiographic Analysis of loosening. Clin. Orthop. 141, 17–27 (1979)

[99] Kaplan, E., Meier, P.: Non parametric estimation form incomplete observations. J. Am. Stat. Assoc. 53, 457 (1958)

[100] Zimmerman, M.C., Buechel, F.F., Pappas, M.J.: Histological Analysis of a Proximally Porous Coated Femoral Hip Stem Implanted For 2 Years. J. Orthop. Rheum. 6, 97–102 (1993)

[101] Yau, S.F.: Three Dimensional Finite Element Analysis of Interfacial Conditions in Porous Coated Femoral Stems. Master's Thesis. New Jersey Institute of Technology (1990)

[102] Clohisy, J.C., Harris, W.H.: Primary hybrid total hip replacement, performed with insertion of the acetabular component without cement and a precoat femoral component with cement: An average ten-year follow-up study. JBJS 81A, 247–255 (1999)

[103] Patel, J., Scott, J.E., Radford, W.J.: Severe polyethylene wear in uncemented acetabular cups system components: a report of 5 cases. J. Arthroplasty 14, 635–636 (1990)

[104] Schrnalzried, T.P., Brown, I.C., Amstutz, H.C., et al.: The role of acetabular component screw holes and/or screws in the development of pelvic osteolysis. In: Proc. Inst. Mech. Eng., vol. 213, pp. 147–153 (1999)

[105] Mihalko, W.M., Papademetriou, T.: Polyethylene liner dissociation with the Harris-Galante II Acetabular Component. Clin. Orthop. 386, 166–172 (2001)

[106] Schulte, K.R., Callaghan, J.J., Kelley, S.S.: The outcome of Charnley Total Hip Arthroplasty with Cement after a minimum Twenty-Year Follow-up. JBJS 75A, 961–975 (1993)

[107] Charnley, J., Cupic, Z.: The nine and ten year results of low friction arthroplasty of the hip. Results using a Survivorship Analysis. Clin. Orthop. 95, 9–25 (1973)

[108] Garellick, G., Malchau, H., Herberts, P.: Survival of hip replacements. A comparison of randomized trial and a registry. Clin. Orthop. 375, 157–167 (2000)

[109] Havinga, M.E., Spruit, M., Anderson, P.G., et al.: Results with the M.E. Muller Cemented, Straight Stem total hip prosthesis. J. of Arthop. 16, 33–36 (2001)

[110] Engh, C.A., Massin, P.: Cementless total hip arthroplasty using The Anatomic Medullary Locking Stem. Clin. Orthop. 249, 141–158 (1989)

[111] Keisu, K.S., Mathiesen, E.B., Lindgren, J.U.: The uncemented fully textured Lord hip prosthesis. Clin. Orthop. 382, 133–142 (2001)

[112] Soyer, J., Avedikian, J., Pries, P., et al.: Long-term outcome of Charnley's femoral implant. A review of 309 cases with follow-up of minimum 20 years. Rev. Chir. Orthop. Reparatrice Appar. Mot. 84, 416–422 (1997)

[113] Cruz-Pardos, A., Garcia-Cimbrelo, E.: The Harris Galante Total Hip Arthroplasty. A minimum 8 year follow up study. J. of Arthop. 16, 586–597 (2001)

[114] Engh, C.A., Glassman, A.H., Suthers, K.E.: The case for porous coated hip implants. Clin. Orthop. 261, 63–81 (1990)

[115] Hozack, W.J., Rothman, R.H., Eng, K., et al.: Primary Cementless Hip Arthroplasty with a Titanium Plasma Spray Prosthesis. Clin. Orthop. 333, 217–225 (1996)

[116] Eingartner, C., Volkmann, R., Winter, E., et al.: Results of an uncemented straight shaft prosthesis after 9 years follow-up. J. of Arthrop. 15, 440–447 (2000)

[117] Head, W.C., Mallory, T.H., Emerson, R.H.: The proximal porous coating alternative for primary total hip arthroplasty. Orthopedics 22, 813–815 (1999)

[118] Owen, T.O., Moran, C.G., Smith, S.R., et al.: Results of Uncemented Porous Coated Anatomic Total Hip replacement. JBJS 76B, 258–262 (1994)

[119] Mallory, T.H., Head, W.C., Lombardi, A.V., et al.: Clinical and radiographical outcome of a cementless, titanium, plasma spray-coated total hip arthroplasty femoral component. J. Arthrop. 11, 653–660 (1996)

[120] Campbell, A.C.L., Rorabeck, C.H., Bourne, R.B., et al.: Thigh Pain after Cementless Hip Arthroplasty, Annoyance or Ill Omen. JBJS 74B, 63–66 (1992)

[121] Buechel, F.F., Pappas, M.J., Greenwald, A.S.: Use of Survivorship and Contact Stress Analyses to Predict the Long-Term Efficacy of New Generation Joint Replacement Designs. A Model for FDA Device Evaluation. Orthop. Rev. 20, 1 (1991)

[122] Jones, V.C., et al.: New Materials for Mobile Bearing Knee Prosthesis - Titanium Nitride Counterface Coatings for Reduction of Polyethylene Wear. In: Hamelynck, K.J., Stiehl, L.B. (eds.) LCS - Mobile Bearing Knee Arthroplasty: 25 Years of Worldwide Experience. ch. 21, Springer, New York (2000)

[123] Black, J.: Biological Performance of Materials; Fundamentals of Biocompatibility, ch.11. Marcel Dekker, New York (1981)

[124] Anderson, K.C., et al.: Post Sintering Heart Treatments to Improve The Mechanical Properties ofTi-6AI-4Va Alloy. In: Transactions of the Twelfth Annual Meeting of The Society for Biomaterials VIII (1986)

[125] Hayashi, K., et al.: Evaluation of Metal Implants Coated with Several Types of Ceramics as Biomaterials. Journal of The Society for Biomaterials 23, 11 (1989)

[126] Cook, S.D., et al.: Cellular Response in Interfacial and Porous Coating Interstitial Tissues of Retrieved Noncemented Components. In: Transactions of the 36th Annual Meeting of the Orthopaedic Research Society, vol. 15, p. 1 (1990)

[127] Kim, K.J., et al.: Comparison of Interface Tissues in Cementless and Cemented Prostheses. In: Transactions of the 36th Annual Meeting of the Orthopaedic Research Society, vol. 23, p. 1 (1990)

[128] Gilbert, J.L., et al.: In vivo Corrosion of Modular Hip Prosthesis Components in Mixed and Similar Metal Combinations. The Effect of Crevice, Stress, Motion, and Alloy Coupling. Journal of Biomedical Materials Research 27 (1993)

[129] Deutschman, A.D., et al.: Machine Design Theory and Practice, ch.7. MacMillan Publishing Co. Inc., New York (1975)

[130] Data on File, Biomedical Engineering Trust (1999)

[131] Gold, B.L., Walker, P.S.: Variables Affecting the Friction and Wear of Metal-on-Plastic Total Hip Joints. Clinical Orthop. and Relocated Res. 100, 270–275 (1975)

[132] Revell, P.A., Weightman, B., Freeman, M.A.R., Roberts, V.B.: The Production and Biology of Polyethylene ear Debris. Arch Orthop. Traum. Surg. 91, 167–181 (1978)

[133] Howmedica, Inc.: BiCentric Endoprosthesis System. Brochure H 1507-2 (1980)

[134] Osteonics Corp. : UHR, Universal Hip Replacement System. Brochure B'R02 (1981)

[135] Mai, K., et al.: Incidence of "Squeaking" After Ceramic-on Ceramic Total Hip Arthroplasty. In: COOR, vol. 468, p. 2 (2009)

[136] Dumbleton, J.H., et al.: The Basis for a Second-Generation Highly Cross-linked UHMWPE. Clin. Orthop. Relat. Res. 453, 265–271 (2006)

[137] Bitsch, R.G., et al.: Reduction of Osteolysis with Use of Marathon Cross-linked Polyethylene. JBJS 90A, 1487–1491 (2008)

[138] Fisher, J., et al.: Tribology of Alternate Bearings. Clin. Orthop. Relat. Res. 453, 24–34 (2006)

[139] Buechel Sr., F.F., Buechel Jr., F.F., Pappas, M.J., D'Alessio, J.: Twenty Year Evaluation of New Jersey LCS Rotating Platform Knee Replacement. The Journal of Knee Surgery 15, 84 (2002)

Chapter 6
The Knee

Abstract. This chapter describes the anatomy, biomechanics and pathology of the knee. The section on anatomy describes the ligamentous structures and musculature. The section on biomechaniics describes tibiofemoral and patellar kinematics as well as forces in the knee. The section on patholgy describes congenital, metabolic, neuromuscular, infectious, autoimmune and post-traumatic pathological conditions. A history of knee relacement is provided. The background of the first, second, third and the most current fourth generation designs is described. The first generation has been largely abandoned but second and third greneration designs are currnently available. These later designs are evaluated for their mechanical and clincal performance. In particular, the charateristics of the currently popular posterior stabilized post-on-cam designs are crticially examined. The extremely high stress in the cam is a highly undesireable charateristic of such designs. Thus, their use in almost all patients seems unwarrented in light of the fact that the forth generation, mobile bearing designs provide the anterior – posterior stability needed. The developement process is given, in detail, for a fourth gereration rotating platform, mobile bearing design. This design, using biological fixation, seems to have potential as a lifetime joint replacement for almost all patients.

6.1 Anatomy

The complex known as the knee joint consists of the femur, tibia, fibula and patella (Fig. 6.1), articulating to accommodate mainly extension and flexion and to a limited degree of varus-valgus and axial rotation.

6.1.1 Ligamentous Structures

The ligamentous structures include the medial collateral ligament (MCL), the lateral collateral ligament (LCL), the anterior cruciate ligament (ACL) and the posterior cruciate ligament (PCL) as illustrated in Fig. 6.2. Additional lateral stabilizers include the popliteus muscle and the ilio-tibial tract (ITT).

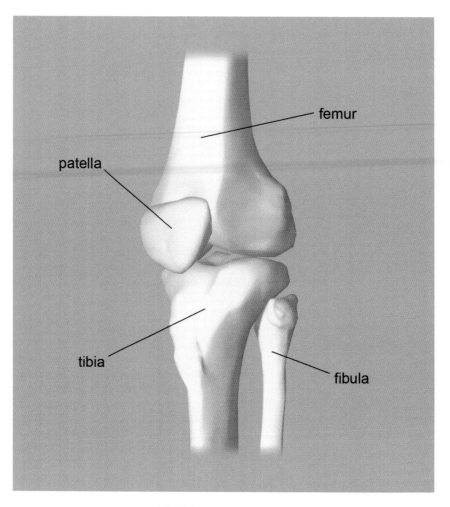

Fig. 6.1 Bones of the Knee.

Additional joint stabilizers and load transfer structures are the medial and lateral menisci, consisting of elastic fibrocartilage. The proximal tibiofibular joint transfers partial lateral loads and allows fibular rotation while connecting the LCL from the lateral femoral epicondyle to the fibular head.

6.1.2 Musculature

The muscles of flexion include the sartorius, gracilis and sartorius which insert on the proximal medial aspect of the tibia as a group known as the pes anserinus (goose foot). The lateral knee flexor is the biceps femoris, which inserts on the fibular head. The medial knee flexor is the semi membranosis which inserts on the posterior proximal tibia. Collectively, the main flexors are known as "hamstrings".

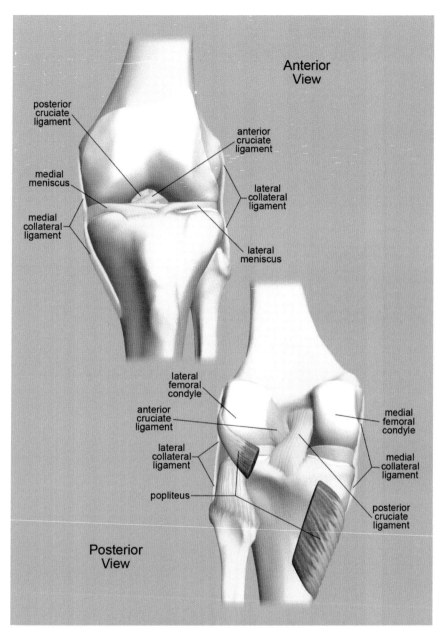

Fig. 6.2 Ligaments of the Knee.

Rotational stabilizers include the popliteus and ITT, as well as contributions from the pes anserinus group. An overview of anterior and posterior knee musculature is represented in Figs 6.3 and 6.4.

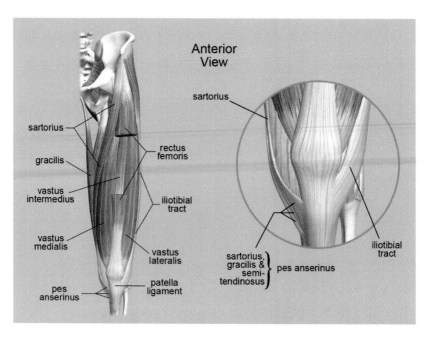

Fig. 6.3 Anterior Knee Musculature.

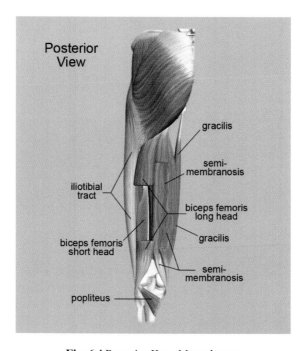

Fig. 6.4 Posterior Knee Musculature.

6.2 Biomechanics

6.2.1 Tibiofemoral Kinematics

The five degrees of freedom associated with the knee joint are illustrated in Fig. 6.5.

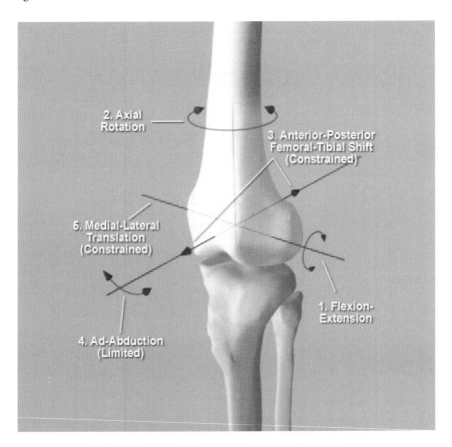

Fig. 6.5 Degrees of Movement and Stability of the Knee.

These are

1. Flexion - Extension; this is the principal motion of the joint.
2. Axial rotation; this motion is limited primarily by the ligaments of the knee.
3. Abduction - Adduction; this motion is limited by the ligaments and the tibiofemoral articulating surfaces.
4. Anterior-posterior (A-P) translation; this motion is limited by the ligaments and the tibiofemoral articulating surfaces.

5.   Medial-Lateral (M-L) translation; this motion is limited by the ligaments and the tibiofemoral articulating surfaces.

The first two are associated with primary knee motion and the remaining with secondary knee motion and stability.

6.2.1.1   Flexion - Extension

The normal passive maximum flexion is typically about 162° and the maximum active flexion is about 135°, as illustrated in Fig. 6.6 [1].

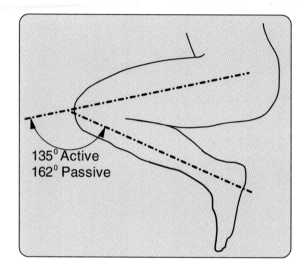

Fig. 6.6 Maximum Flexion in the Normal Knee.

Any restriction of this motion is undesirable as it adversely affects knee function and can produce undesirable loading on the prosthesis, ligaments and bone fixation interface.

6.2.1.2   Axial Rotation

At full extension the "screw home" action of the cruciates prevents significant axial rotation. As the knee is flexed, however, these ligaments allow this motion.

Normal maximum rotation is about 30° at 90° of flexion (Fig. 6.7). Such rotation can occur during normal human activities, such as arising from a chair. During walking, axial rotation is about ± 6°, as illustrated in Fig. 6.8 and during deep flexion about 20° [1, 2].

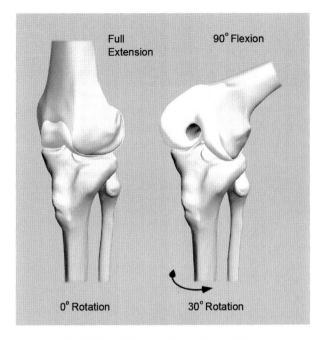

Fig. 6.7 Axial Rotation in the Normal Knee.

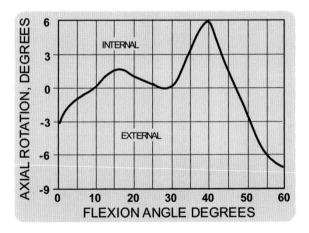

Fig. 6.8 Axial Rotation vs. Flexion during Walking.

6.2.2 Stability and Secondary Motion

The normal knee joint is stable and, thus, is constrained against significant ab-adduction, anterior-posterior and medial-lateral motion although some secondary ab-adduction and A-P motion is normal.

There are two types of stability. Intrinsic stability provided by the shape of the articulating surfaces and extrinsic stability provided by soft tissues. All except M-L stability is essentially extrinsic.

6.2.2.1   Abduction - Adduction Stability and Motion

Such motion is normal during many human activities. The abduction, or lifting of the lateral condyle, occurs in the swing phase of normal walking and is about 8° as shown in Fig. 6.9 [2].

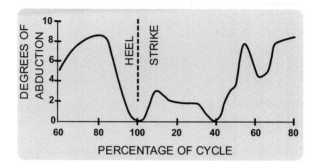

Fig. 6.9 Abduction during Walking.

Valgus – varus stability is primarily extrinsic. The action of the ligaments in providing this stability is illustrated in Fig. 6.10.

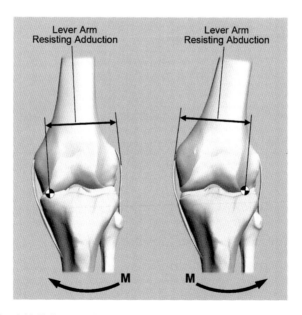

Fig. 6.10 Collateral Ligament Lever Arms Resisting Ab-Adduction.

The cruciate ligaments also play a part in providing varus-valgus stability [3] but primarily provide A-P and rotational stability.

6.2.2.2   Anterior - Posterior Stability and Translation

Roll back of the femur on the tibial plateau during flexion is an important characteristic of the knee joint. It is produced by the action of the posterior cruciate and the shape of the articulating surfaces as shown in Fig. 6.11.

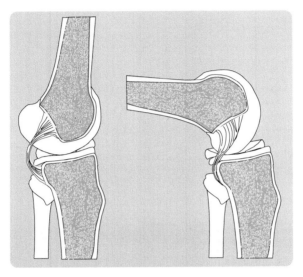

Fig. 6.11 Posterior Cruciate Tightens on Flexion Producing Rollback of the Femur on the Tibia.

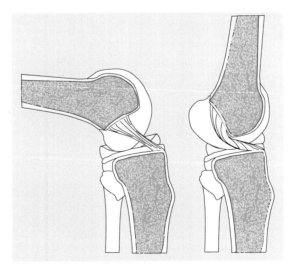

Fig. 6.12 Anterior Cruciate Tightens Causing Forward Roll of the Femur on the Tibia.

Roll forward during extension is produced by the anterior cruciate as illustrated in Fig. 6.12.

Roll back on the more congruent medial condyle is about 5mm while the roll back on the relatively incongruent lateral condyle is about 15mm as illustrated in Fig. 6.13 [4].

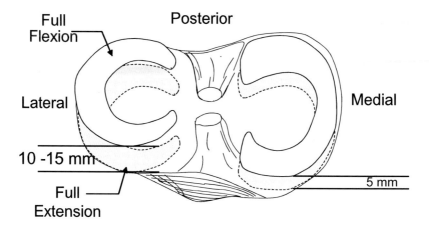

Fig. 6.13 Movement of the Menisci during Flexion and Extension.

Roll back improves the function of the quadriceps by increasing the quadriceps lever arm in flexion, where greater leverage is needed. This is illustrated in Fig. 6.14 [5].

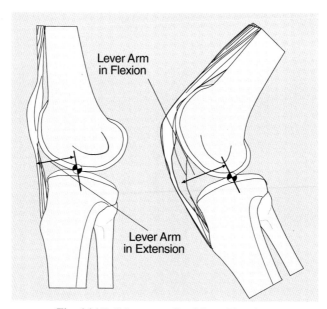

Fig. 6.14 Roll Improves Quadriceps Function.

The cruciate ligaments act in concert to produce predictable A-P translation while also maintaining A-P stability. The disruption of the cruciate ligaments disrupts the normal roll back/roll forward A-P translation function making anterior-posterior motion unpredictable and disrupting A-P stability.

The ligaments adapt to the natural geometry of the articulating surfaces of the knee. Since the tibial plane is inclined posteriorly [6], the ligaments accommodate A-P, or roll back, motion along this posteriorly inclined plane as illustrated in Fig. 6.15.

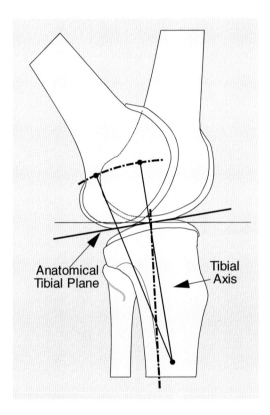

Fig. 6.15 Normal Collateral Ligament Motion Pattern.

6.2.2.3 Medial-Lateral

M-L stability under load bearing is primarily intrinsic. The ligaments, of course, also play a role. M-L motion is inhibited by the Tibial Spine and the resistance of the ligaments as illustrated in Fig. 6.16.

There is, however, about 2mm of M-L motion in the normal knee [4, 5].

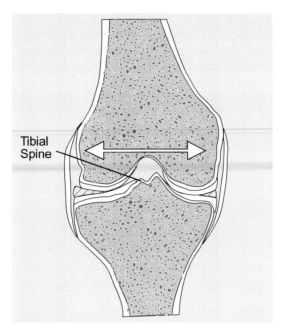

Fig. 6.16 M-L Stability Provided by the Tibial Spine.

6.2.3   Patellofemoral Kinematics

6.2.3.1   Patellofemoral Motion

a) Patellofemoral Tracking

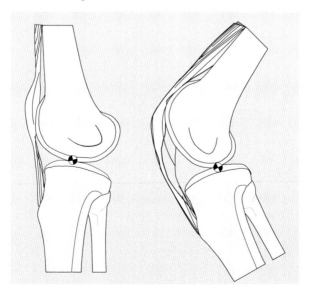

Fig. 6.17 Tracking of the Patella during Knee Flexion.

b) Axial Rotation

The axial rotation of the tibia with respect to the femur produces a medial-lateral excursion of the patella tendon insertion. This results in axial rotation of the patella relative to the femur as illustrated in Fig. 6.18.

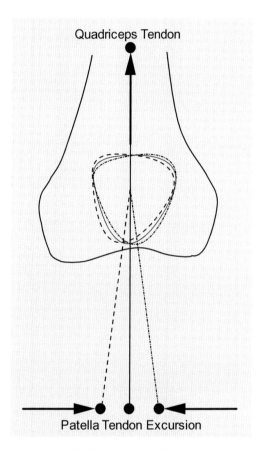

Fig. 6.18 Axial Rotation of the Patella.

Rotation during walking is about 6° of internal rotation and 8° of external rotation as shown in Fig. 6.19. Rotation can be more than double these amounts for other activities [2].

The patella does not articulate with the sulcus of the femur until about 45° of flexion. Due to the oblique pull of the quadriceps, the patella tends to have a lateral tilt until about 45° of flexion where the compressive loads are sufficiently great to force contact with the femur on both its lateral and medial middle facets.

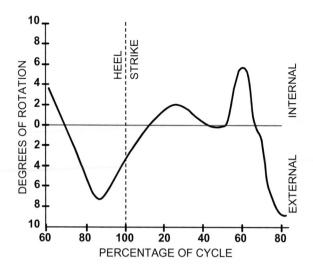

Fig. 6.19 Patellar Rotation During Walking.

6.2.3.2 Patellofemoral Stability

The patella is maintained in the sulcus of the anterior femur by the shape of their articulating surfaces and the pull of the quadriceps. This pull, however, has a significant lateral component and can produce patellar subluxation, particularly in women.

6.2.4 Forces

6.2.4.1 Tibiofemoral Loading

The forces in the knee during walking are of the order of about 3 to 4 times body weight in normal gait as shown in Fig. 6.20 [7].

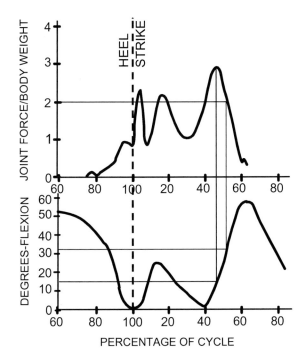

Fig. 6.20 Tibiofemoral Joint Forces and Motion for Normal Gait.

Peak forces occur at about 20° of flexion but substantial forces are present from 0° to 40° as shown in Fig. 6.20. As may be seen from Fig. 6.21 the loading is not equally shared by the condyles. Rather, the bulk of the loading in the high loading phase occurs in the more congruent medial condyle which carries twice the maximum load of the lateral condyle. This high loading phase is accompanied by significant lateral collateral ligament loading and abduction. The less congruent lateral condyle is more highly loaded during the lightly loaded swing phase.

Thus the knee experiences an oscillating varus-valgus loading which makes tibial fixation difficult.

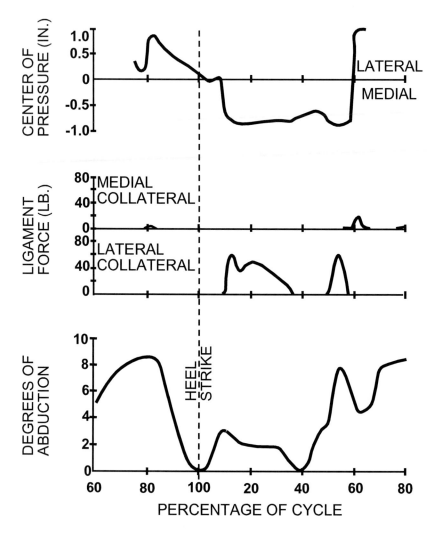

Fig. 6.21 Oscillation of Knee Forces and Their Effect on Condylar Loading, Ligaments and Abduction.

6.2.4.2   Patellofemoral Loading

At low flexion angles loading of the patella is relatively low as illustrated in Fig. 6.22.

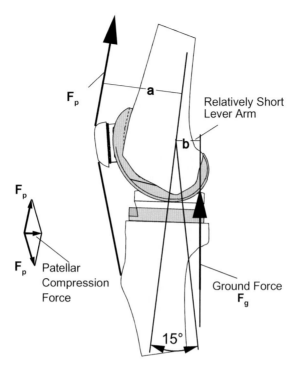

Fig. 6.22 Patellar Forces at Low Flexion Angles.

Since

$$F_p = b \times F_g / a \tag{1}$$

the lever arm **b** associated with the ground reaction force F_g is small, the patellar tendon tension F_p is small, and since the angle between the patella and quadriceps tendon tension vectors are only slightly misaligned at low flexion angles and the patellar compression force, which is the vector sum of the tendon vectors, is small in comparison to the tendon vectors. The patellar compression force is, therefore, doubly small.

The patellar forces are, however, quite large in flexion as illustrated in Fig. 6.23.

Here the ground force lever arm **b'** is relatively large resulting in relatively large quadriceps and patellar tendon forces. Further, since the forces are more misaligned, the patellar compression force is larger than the tendon forces at large flexion angles. The patellar compression forces are estimated to be 111N (25 lbs) at 15° (walking), 1557N (347 lbs) at 30° (stair ascent) and 4003N (893 lbs) at 110° of flexion (knee bends) [8].

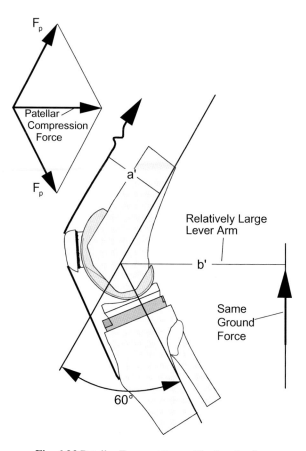

Fig. 6.23 Patellar Forces at Large Flexion Angles.

6.3 Pathology

Disease processes involving the knee joint are usually classified into congenital, metabolic, neuro-muscular, infectious, autoimmune and post-traumatic.

6.3.1 Congenital

Incomplete or poor embryonic development of the knee can result from congenital anomalies such as hypoplastic patellae or discoid menisci, which can lead to poor knee function, degenerative joint disease or maltracking of the extensor mechanism. Surgical correction of malalignment, instability or maltracking of the extensor mechanism may be necessary to allow restoration of function.

6.3.2 Metabolic

Bone disorders involving deficiencies in calcium metabolism secondary to hormonal, genetic or nutritional imbalance can affect the integrity of the bones and ligaments of the knee, leading to joint destruction or malalignment. Such disorders need to be accurately diagnosed and treated with appropriate medical management in addition to consideration of possible arthroscopy for internal derangement and corrective osteotomies for extraarticular malalignment problems.

6.3.3 Neuromuscular

Diseases affecting the nerves and muscles of the knee can cause significant gait disturbances and instability problems. Lumbar disc disease can have a seriously disabling effect on quadriceps and hamstring function if L_3, L_4 and L_5 nerve roots are affected. Other neurological conditions that impair the motor function of the knee or allow "back-knee" deformities essentially disable a patient from meaningful ambulation activities without walking aids. Without stability and motor function, knee fusion becomes a reasonable but drastic alternative to provide lower limb function.

6.3.4 Infectious

Sepsis of the knee from any gram positive or gram negative bacteria can result in destruction of the knee joint, known as septic arthritis. These joints are at significant risk of re-infection, but knee fusion is so disabling that multiple attempts at curing an infection using antibiotic impregnated bone cement is often attempted, as long as a functioning extensor mechanism is available and ligamentous stability can be achieved or substituted during knee replacement surgery. Knee fusion or resection arthroplasty are last resort options in the case of persistent knee joint infections.

6.3.5 Autoimmune

Arthritis of the knee can be a result of autoimmune disorders such as rheumatoid or psoriatic arthritis, where the body perceives a foreign antigen to be present, requiring neutralization by host defenses, even though they are not foreign, but in fact, are the normal cartilage structure of the host. In the normal defense process, the host destroys its own normal cartilage by mistake. Evidence suggests that osteoarthritis has a genetic component that may be related to an autoimmune phenomenon as well. In any event, these arthritic conditions have a similar end-stage pathology, which makes them suitable candidates for joint replacement to improve their function.

6.3.6 Post-Traumatic

Fractures, dislocations or severe ligament injuries can compromise knee joint function and in many cases cause severe cartilage destruction, similar to osteoarthritis. In patients with correctable deformities, reconstructable ligaments and a functioning extensor mechanism, knee joint replacement offers an excellent functional alternative to disabling pain and deformity [9].   An x-ray of post-traumatic knee arthritis is seen in Fig. 6.24.

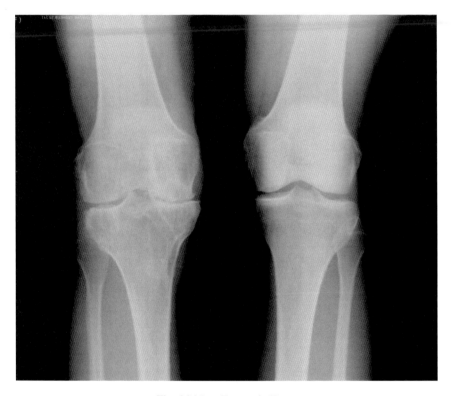

Fig. 6.24 Post Traumatic Knee.

6.4 Knee Replacement

6.4.1 First Generation Designs

Early hinge designs of the 1950's, such as the "Waldius" and later the "GUEPAR" knees restricted motion to a single flexion-extension axis. Although they initially worked reasonably well, when they were simply press-fit into the bone, they showed early loosening when used with cement. This loosening is attributed to over-constraint resulting from lack of axial and ad-abduction rotation producing large axial and varus-valgus torques [10, 11] as illustrated in Fig. 6.25.

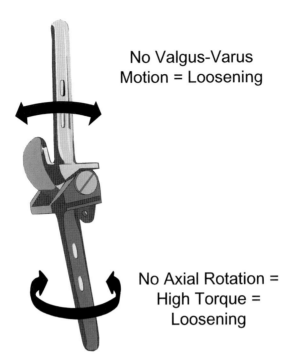

No Valgus-Varus Motion = Loosening

No Axial Rotation = High Torque = Loosening

Fig. 6.25 Loosening Resulting from Lack of Axial Rotation in Hinge Type Knees.

Later resurfacing designs of the late 60's, such as the "Geomedic" and "Geometric", also rapidly failed due to lack of axial rotation, as shown in Fig. 6.26 and lack of provision for roll back [12, 13] as illustrated in Fig. 6.27.

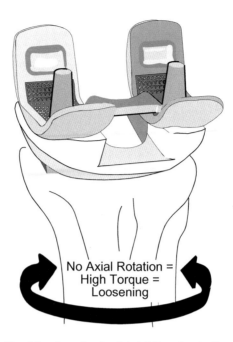

Fig. 6.26 Loosening Resulting from Lack of Axial Rotation in Resurfacing Knees of the "Geomedic" Type.

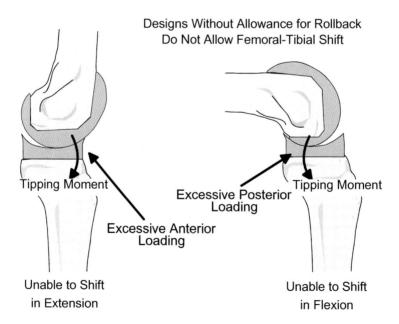

Fig. 6.27 Excessive Anterior-Posterior Tipping Forces Resulting from Lack of Provision for Roll Back.

Less constrained designs such as the "Marmor" and "Gunston" designs of the late 60's failed due to excessive contact stress and material overloading [14, 15] as shown in Fig. 6.28.

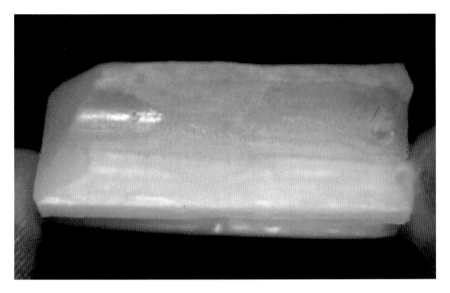

Fig. 6.28 Worn Gunston Tibial Component.

None of the first generation resurfacing designs had provision for patellar replacement.

6.4.2   Second Generation Designs

The 1970's saw the introduction of improved resurfacing designs which provided for patellar replacement. The "Total Condylar" and "Townley" designs worked reasonably well. The principal problems were; lack of adequate flexion, patellar wear and loosening, posterior subluxation of the Total Condylar and tibial loosening and excessive pitting type wear with both devices [16-20]. Tibial loosening problems resulted in the introduction of metal-backed bearings, which dominate the market today.

Attempts were made to develop hinge designs with axial rotation. The "Spherocentric" knee, illustrated in Fig. 6.29, provided axial rotation and even some varus-valgus motion.

Failure of this design was, however quite rapid [21] due to loosening which was the result of varus-valgus constraint combined with excessive bone removal and inadequate stem fixation.

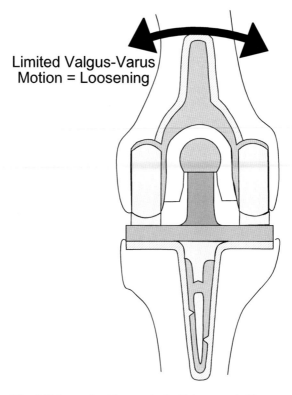

Fig. 6.29 Loosening Torques in the Spherocentric Knee.

Problems of subluxation of the Total Condylar knee design led to the introduction of a posterior stabilized version [19] in which a post on the bearing acting in concert with a cam on the femoral component provided added A-P stability and some roll back in deep flexion. Variations of this design quickly proliferated and they are the most widely used knee replacement type used today.

6.4.3   Third Generation Designs

The mid, and late, 1970's saw the introduction of mobile bearing knee designs, such as the "Oxford" [23] and "New Jersey LCS" [24] knees. These designs provide mobility and congruency by use of a second bearing surface articulating against a metal tibial platform. The mobile bearing concept solved the dilemma of congruency vs. constraint facing knee designers of the time as illustrated in Fig. 6.30.

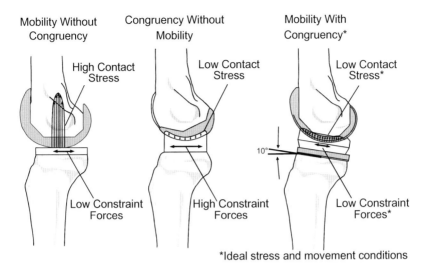

Mobility Without Congruency — High Contact Stress — Low Constraint Forces

Congruency Without Mobility — Low Contact Stress — High Constraint Forces

Mobility With Congruency* — Low Contact Stress* — 10° — Low Constraint Forces*

*Ideal stress and movement conditions

Fig. 6.30 Mobile Bearing Solution to the Dilemma of Mobility vs Congruity.

6.4.3.1 The Oxford Knee

The "Oxford" knee Developed by Goodfellow and O'Connor starting in 1976 was the first mobile bearing knee and possibly the first mobile bearing joint replacement in the world [23].

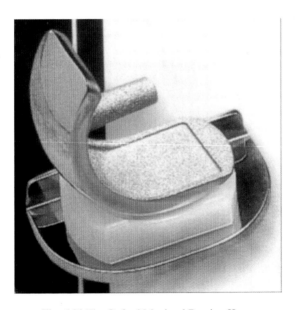

Fig. 6.31 The Oxford Meniscal Bearing Knee.

6.4.3.2 The Noiles Hinge Knee

Noiles [25] developed the concepts of a rotating hinge in 1977. A number of iterations of his original design were subsequently developed and are still being sold today.

6.4.3.3 The LCS Knee

The New Jersey LCS Knee System [26, 27], illustrated in Fig. 6.32, was originally developed during the period from 1977 through 1985. It is the first, FDA approved knee replacement available and only one of few approved systems available today in the United States of America. The system has been in highly successful clinical use for more than thirty years and is approved for use by the FDA after their evaluation of extensive, well controlled, clinical studies [28-32].

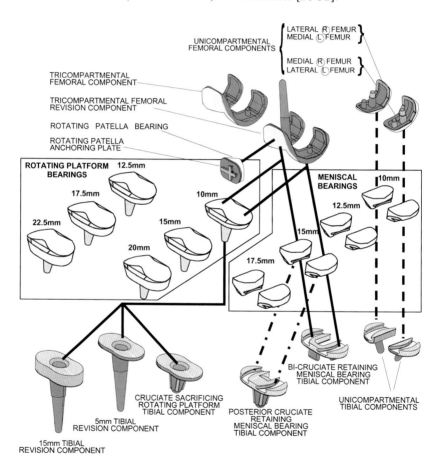

Fig. 6.32 New Jersey Mark II LCS Knee System.

The meniscal bearing, Posterior Retaining Tibial Platform was replaced by the A-P Glide Platform about 1997. This later device substituted a single meniscal bearing for the twin bearings of the original and uses the Rotating Platform Tibial Component and a Control Arm to permit axial rotation and A-P translation of the bearing [33].

6.4.3.4 Others

During the 1990's additional mobile bearing designs were introduced by most manufacturers that marketed knee replacement systems in Europe. These include the Zimmer MBK, Howmedica's Interax ISA, J& J's PFC Sigma RP, Sulzer SAL and others [34-37]. None of these introduced anything new of significance.

Also introduced was an inappropriate version of the PFC Sigma RPF posterior stabilized Rotating Platform knee which substituted an unneeded post and cam for needed tibiofemoral congruity [78].

6.4.4 The Fourth Generation

Experience with the LCS and the improved availability of materials and manufacturing process provided information to allow further development and refinement of the LCS, or Buechel - Pappas Mark II mobile bearing knee replacement. A series of new designs were then developed during the period from 1998 through 2009 leading to the B-P Mark V Total Knee Replacement shown in Fig. 6.33.

The metallic components of this knee are made of wrought titanium alloy coated with a wear and scratch resistant TiN ceramic coating described earlier. Co-Cr versions are available as well. The articulating surfaces have been refined so that the peak contact stress in the Mark V is about half that of the very successful LCS.

These knees implants are manufactured and distributed worldwide by Endotec, Inc. of Orlando, Florida and TKK Health Care of Chennai, India.

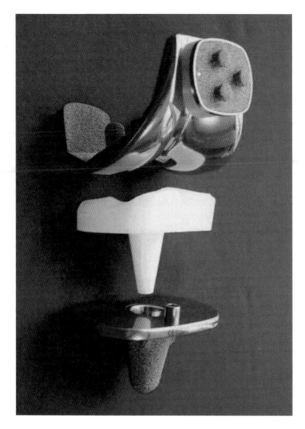

Fig. 6.33 The B-P Mark V total Knee Replacement.

6.5 Design Evaluation

The primary lessons of these early designs are:

a) Avoid unnecessary prosthetic constraints where possible. Allow the soft tissue constraints to act. If the soft tissue constraints are not available and prosthetic constraints must be used, provide sufficient fixation to resist the expected loading resulting from these constraints.

b) Accommodate normal knee motion and loading. Failure to provide for normal knee motion and loading can produce excessive stresses in the prosthesis and at the bone-prosthesis interface.

c) Mobile bearings are needed to provide the necessary degree of congruity and mobility to provide a long service life using materials currently available for knee prostheses.

d) The design of a successful knee replacement is complex and careful design is necessary to avoid serious design defects.

The generally poor performance of the second generation knees is typified by the PCA device, which, at one time, was the most widely used knee replacement. Its clinical performance is shown in Fig. 6.34. Failure was due to excessive contact stress [39].

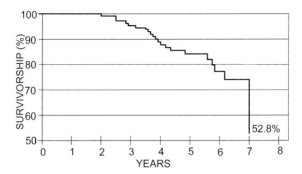

Fig. 6.34 Survivorship of 108 Cementless PCA Knees.

These lessons were available to all by the end of the 1970's and yet no substantial new developments in knee design have occurred since then. The New Jersey LCS and its derivatives document the successful application of these principles to tricompartmental knees.

6.5.1 Second Generation Designs

6.5.1.1 Posterior Stabilized (PS) Knee Replacements

a) Introduction
Posterior stabilized knee designs are among the most popular type of knee replacement systems. Insall and Burstein first introduced such a design in 1982 to reduce the tendency towards posterior dislocation of the Total Condylar knee introduced some years earlier. This approach apparently solved the problem effectively [19, 40-43]. Further, the claim that forced roll back of the femur relative to the tibia improves quadriceps function has theoretical merit. Such improvement is, however, difficult to show clinically [44]. Many imitations and modifications have followed [45, 46].

Still, as is common in design innovation, advantages are often partially offset by disadvantages associated with a given design approach. Thus, one sees reports of excessive wear and fracture of stabilizing posts [47-55]. Pulaski et al [52] found damage on all of the 23 posts they examined and seven (30%) of the posts "exhibited severe damage with gross loss of polyethylene". Furman et al [55] in a study of 234 Insall – Burstein (IB) PS I and PS II bearing inserts found "severe wear" in 25% of the IB PS I inserts and 38% of the IB PS II inserts. Such damage is the expected result of the excessive contact stresses reported by Akasagi et al [56] and Morra and Greenwald [57].

The femoral recess used to house the tibial post and to clear the post on implantation of the femoral component also produces problems with the patella [58-62], bone loss with resulting fractures [63] and component tissue entrapment [64]. This recess also eliminates a substantial part of the femoral surface against which the patella articulates and thus may increase patellofemoral contact stresses in flexion. Furthermore, restriction in axial rotation of such devices may contribute to tibial loosening [65].

Early to mid-term evaluation of rotating-platform designs with intercondylar posts have demonstrated painful patella-femoral crepitus also known as "patellar clunk" in 5-13% of patients [66-68]. These patients require surgery to remove the fibrous nodules that develop on the quadriceps tendon that result from "snapping" across the open intercondylar box of the femoral component rather than maintaining a smooth similar articulation throughout flexion as seen in conventional rotating platform designs with a "patella friendly" intercondylar surface. Additionally, the use of the extra bony resection to introduce the intercondylar box in the femur also predisposes to condylar fractures in very small patients due to a stress riser effect in compromised bone. These factors would mitigate against the use of these devices, especially since conventional rotating platforms with central rotation pegs have demonstrated substantially lower contact stresses [69] and equivalent or superior range of motion to the intercondylar post variants over the long term [35, 70].

Several sources discuss tibiofemoral and patellofemoral contact stresses in congruent and incongruent articulations [71-73]. As a class, PS knees need to give up congruity if they are to provide roll back without substantially increasing post to cam stresses.

Long-term clinical experience with a well designed surgical approach and implant seems to show that posterior stabilization by means of cam and post may not be needed for controlling posterior dislocation in most patients [28, 74-77]. Further, in comparing the results of Kim [70] with those of Ranawat et al [78] there seems to be no added flexion provided by a PS design over a well-designed rotating platform knee replacement. Thus, a question arises as to where the use of a PS knee replacement is justified in light of the problems associated with them. In other words, what are the clinical risks versus the clinical benefits associated with PS knee designs?

It is useful, therefore, to consider in detail the mechanical performance characteristics of posterior stabilized designs and to compare their properties. Such a comparison will allow one to better understand, where, and to what degree, posterior stabilized designs may be clinically useful.

b) Methods and Materials

Seven PS type knee implants are compared. Of these, six are fixed tibial bearing devices and one is a mobile bearing design. Four of the fixed bearing types are conventional cam and post designs similar to the original Insall – Burstein (IB) device. Two, the Kinemax and Maxim, are early engagement post and cam devices. In addition, a PS version of the LCS [79] using a conventional post and cam, but with a rotating bearing is evaluated. Also evaluated is the LCS Rotating

Bearing knee to allow a comparison of posterior stabilized and conventional designs. Except for the LCS based, PFC Sigma [35], NexGen LCCK and Maxim knees, where drawings were available, the detailed configuration of the devices was determined by measurements on retrieved implants using a Brown and Sharp Microval three-dimensional coordinate measuring machine.

The devices are normalized for size by scaling the devices so that the A/P dimension of each is 62mm. This allows a comparison of equally sized devices and thus avoids the effect of size variation. The functional and wear related properties were evaluated. The following are evaluated and compared:

1. Maximum device flexion and angle of flexion at which roll back begins:

Maximum flexion is defined as the largest flexion angle that can be produced with engagement of the femoral and tibial articulating surfaces and with avoidance of edge, or other grossly incongruent, contact. Initiation of roll back is the flexion angle at which contact between the posterior stabilizing elements first occurs. Zero flexion is considered the orientation where the distal femoral fixation surface is parallel to the bottom of the tibial tray.

2. The maximum allowable axial rotation at 15°, 60°, 90° and 120° of flexion:

Maximum axial rotation is defined as the rotation from the neutral position where impingement of the edges of the post and cam first occurs or until the tibiofemoral articulating surfaces disengage and edge contact occurs, whichever is least.

3. The femoral roll back at 15°, 30°, 45°, 60°, 90° 105°, 120° and 135° of flexion:

Femoral roll back is defined as the posterior translation of the center of contact of the femur on the tibia from a position where the femoral component would contact the thinnest portion of the bearing (the low point) to the femoral component center of contact position produced by the cam to post interaction as illustrated in Fig. 6.35.

4. The estimated quadriceps lever arm at these flexion angles:

The lever arm is the distance from the estimated instant, two dimensional, center of rotation of the tibia relative to the femur to the patellar tendon. This property is illustrated in Fig. 6.35.

5. The dislocation height at these flexion angles:

Dislocation height is defined as the displacement normal to the natural tibial condylar surface that will lift one of the stabilizing members above the other thus allowing posterior dislocation. It is the greater of the post or articular surface dislocation heights. This property is also illustrated in Fig. 6.35.

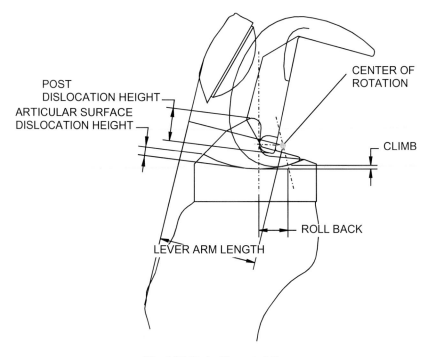

Fig. 6.35 Study Characteristics.

It should be noted that the tibial condylar surface is not perpendicular to the tibial axis. Rather it is inclined posteriorly about approximately 7° [6]. Thus, the ligaments adapt to such an inclined surface with regard to controlling tibiofemoral motion. Further joint forces are essentially perpendicular to the tibial condylar surface in order to avoid unnecessary shearing forces on the knee. The implantation of a tibial component perpendicular to the axis of the tibia creates unnecessary shearing forces and reduces dislocation height.

6.   The post to cam peak contact stresses at 75°, 105° and 135° of flexion where most post to cam contact occurs.

Axial rotation is taken as zero in the determination of these stresses. A 2000 N compressive force perpendicular to the tibial resection plane is applied to the femoral component. In addition, a 500 N shear force, perpendicular to the compressive force, is used to load the post against cam. [80] This shear force is used by Akasagi et al [56] for their contact stress studies.

Here the joint reaction force is assumed perpendicular to the natural tibial condylar surface. The compression force on the bearings, however, must be essentially perpendicular to the tangent to the bearing articular surface at the point of contact. Thus, a shear force must be introduced to produce a resulting perpendicular joint compression force. Where the tibial component is not implanted with a normal posterior inclination additional shear is introduced increasing the post contact stresses. Further, where the femoral component climbs "up hill" [81] on the tibial bearing on roll back the compressive force adds an additional shear force on the stabilization elements further increasing contact stresses. The effect of tibial component inclination and climb are considered in this analysis.

The contact stress computations are performed using classical elasticity methods from applied mechanics given in Refs. [73, 82 and 83] to estimate the peak contact stresses. Line contact stresses were computed using the simple Herzian equations for cylinders in contact [82] for the devices having cam to post line contact. The method of Ref. [83], for point contact, is used for the PFC Sigma and Maeva knees. An elastic modulus of 614 MPa, which is the modulus of UHMWPe at body temperature [84], is used for the bearing stiffness. The peak stress is the critical stress producing the worst damage.

Stresses near and beyond the yield strength of the UHMWPe will be overestimated by linear analysis. Linear values in excess of the yield strength are, however, to be avoided. If linear analysis determines a value of peak stress greater than the yield strength, the design is not satisfactory. Further, the amount that the value is in excess of the yield is indicative as to the amount and speed of the yielding and damage that will occur. Thus, linear values can be quite useful in comparisons.

This data is used to generate tables and graphs that compare the performance of the devices. In addition retrieved specimens are examined and analyzed to compare clinical performance with performance expected on the basis of the characteristics associated with typical PS knee designs evaluated.

c) Results
As may be seen in Table 6.1 none of the devices permits a maximum normal passive flexion of 162° [1]. Most of the fixed bearing cam and post designs fail to mechanically provide normal, maximum active flexion of 135° [1].

Table 6.1 Maximum Flexion and Flexion Angle in Degrees at Initiation of Roll back.

Implant	Maximum	Roll back Initiation	Comments
IB PS II	113	69	Relatively congruent fixed Bearing
Maeva	125	76	Initial 8 mm posterior femoral position
NexGen PS	115	68	Posterior femoral position - No significant roll back
PFC Sigma	119	68	Moderately incongruent theoretical point cam contact
Kinemax	126	60	Initial 5.3mm anterior femoral position
Maxim	139	15	Early engagement may produced increased wear
LCS-PS	144	75	Rotating Platform Bearing
LCS	155	~	Conventional Rotating Platform Bearing

Further, it may be seen that with the exception of the Maxim knees initiation of roll back, as illustrated in Fig. 6.36, occurs relatively late thereby losing roll back properties in important activities such as stair climbing.

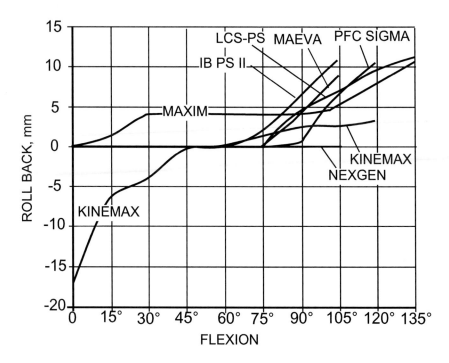

Fig. 6.36 Roll Back in mm as a Function of Flexion Angle.

Table 6.2 demonstrates that the axial rotation in all designs, other than the LCS-PS knee, is far below the normal maximum axial rotation of at least 20° that is needed in deep flexion [1]. Most provide marginally sufficient axial rotation to accommodate walking. In some cases, there is insufficient axial rotation to accommodate expected surgical misalignment.

Table 6.2 Axial Rotation in Degrees vs. Flexion Angle.

Implant	15°	60°	90°	120°	Comments
IB PS II	7	6	5	~	Inadequate, particularly in deep flexion
Maeva	2	11	2	2	Roll back results in loss of T/F contact on rotation
NexGen PS	7	6	5	~	Inadequate, particularly in deep flexion
PFC Sigma	4	4	4	4	Inadequate axial rotation
Kinemax	4	4	8	8	Inadequate axial rotation
Maxim	4	4	8	8	Inadequate axial rotation
LCS-PS	360	360	360	360	Unrestricted Axial Rotation
LCS	360	360	360	360	Unrestricted Axial Rotation

Except for those devices such as the LCS-PS, PFC Sigma and the Maeva which provide for axial rotation, the actual contact stresses resulting from the corner edge contact between the post and cam resulting from axial rotation, would be significantly higher than those estimated for line contact at zero axial rotation. Thus, axial rotation greatly magnifies the already excessive stresses observed at zero degrees.

Most devices do not provide significant roll back until more than 75° of flexion is achieved. Thus, they provide little advantage for stair climbing and descent.

It should be noted that at zero flexion the Kinemax produces an anterior position of the femoral component on the bearing resulting in a reduction in the quadriceps lever arm at full extension. Further this anterior positioning results in an anterior climb of 2.3mm resulting in a reduction in the prosthetic gap on flexion producing loosening of ligament tension.

More important than roll back in improving quadriceps function is an increase in the quadriceps lever arm resulting from roll back. This property is shown in Fig. 6.37. It may be seen that the largest lever arm is provided by the NexGen PS knee even though that device does not provide any significant roll back as shown in Fig. 6.36.

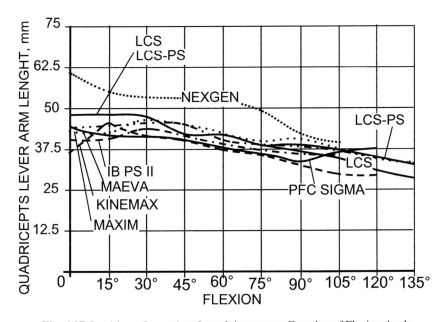

Fig. 6.37 Quadriceps Lever Arm Length in mm as a Function of Flexion Angle.

The LCS-PS and IB PS II provide similar lever arm lengths even though the LCS fails to provide roll back. Comparing the LCS conventional knee with the LCS-PS, however, it may be seen that roll back can increase the lever arm in deep flexion.

It should be noted that, since in deep flexion, most devices, including the LCS, allow anterior – posterior translation the true lever arm will depend on the action of the quadriceps and hamstring muscles and on posterior soft tissue impingement. Thus, for example, quadriceps pull or posterior impingement of the tibia, or tibial component, with the posterior soft tissues may produce an anterior translation of the tibial relative to the femur thus, increasing the effective quadriceps lever arm length. Thus, it is not clear that cam – to - post forced roll back is, in fact, advantageous.

Fig. 6.38 shows that at low flexion angles some of the devices provide little posterior stabilization. Thus, dislocation can be a problem with such PS designs [85, 86]. It should be noted the current LCS provides 8.5 mm of dislocation height for its entire range of motion due to the conformity of its articulating surfaces.

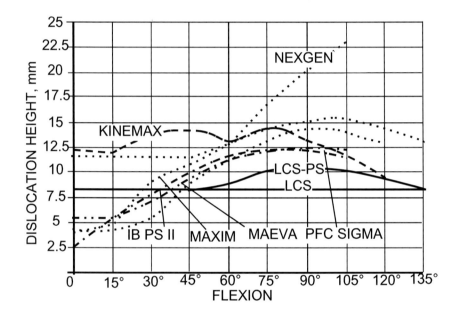

Fig. 6.38 Dislocation Height in mm as a Function of Flexion Angle.

As may be seen from Fig. 6.39 all the PS knees have post contact stresses greatly in excess of the manufacturer's acceptable limit of l0Mpa [84]. Such stresses are unacceptable by accepted design engineering standards [82]. Post stresses often exceed the estimated yield stress of the UHMWPe in compression [73]. In such cases rapid degeneration of the post is expected and is well documented [48-54].

That axial rotation will produce edge contact at the corners of the post face in fixed bearing designs greatly increasing contact stresses at these points may be seen from Figures 6.40 and 6.41. Here wear is seen as "wrapped" around these corners. Thus, the stresses of Fig. 6.39 do not adequately reflect the seriousness of the overload of fixed bearing post designs.

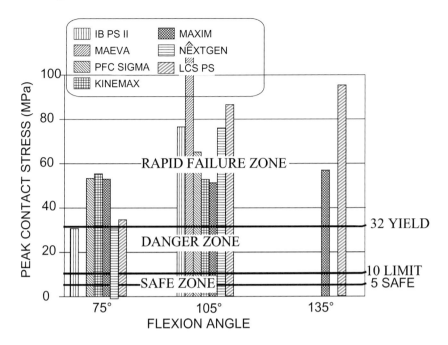

Fig. 6.39 Cam against Post Peak Contact Stresses vs. Flexion Angle.

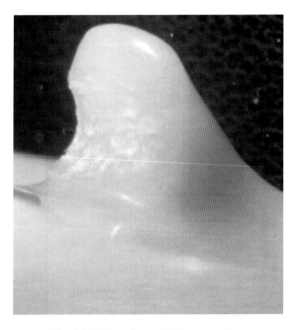

Fig. 6.40 "Wrap Around" Wear on a Post.

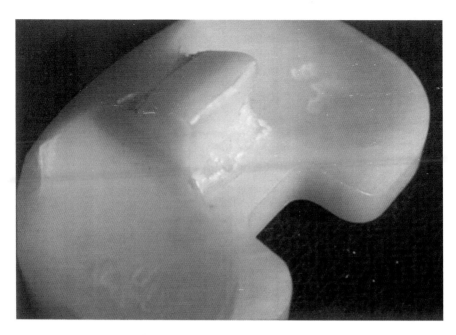

Fig. 6.41 Tibial Post and Bearing Wear.

Fig. 6.41 shows an example of both anterior and posterior post damage as well as damage to the tibiofemoral articulation surfaces. Banks, Harmon and Hodge [47] report anterior post damage as do references [88, 89]. Anterior post damage can be substantial as may be seen in Fig. 6.42.

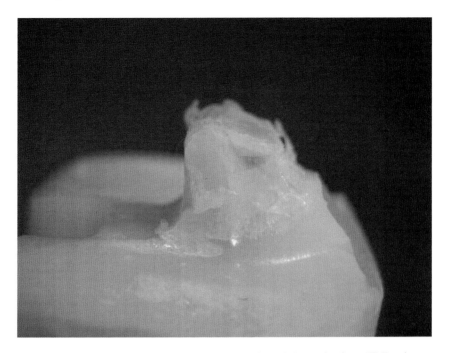

Fig. 6.42 Tibial Post Damage Due to Restriction in Axial Rotation in an IB Bearing.

Fig. 6.42 also shows post damage that is apparently the result of impingement associated with both axial rotation and valgus/varus tilt of the device. Examining the base of the post in Fig. 6.41, one may also observe the effect of axial rotation producing the greater wear near the corners. Such damage is expected considering the excessive contact stress and lack of accommodation for axial rotation, hyperextension and lateral load resistance during varus/valgus motion in most designs.

Figure 6.43 shows the superior view of the bearing of Fig. 6.42. Here again it may be seen the post damage exceeds the damage to the tibiofemoral articulation surfaces. It is probably fortunate that cam – to - post engagement occurs at relatively large flexion angles. Thus, frequent activities such as stair climbing do not produce cam to post contact and the resulting wear. Contact occurs on relatively infrequent activities, such as arising from a chair where, since the patient's arms often assist in such action, knee loading may be relatively low.

From Figures 6.40-6.43 it may be seen that post damage, which results from relatively infrequent activities, is greater than tibiofemoral articulation surface damage that results from much more frequent activities. Evidence of this less frequent engagement may be seen in Fig. 6.43 where the posterior tibial bearing surface, which is articulating with the femoral component, has relatively low wear. This greater wear at less frequent contact is the result of the much greater contact stresses associated with cam to post contact.

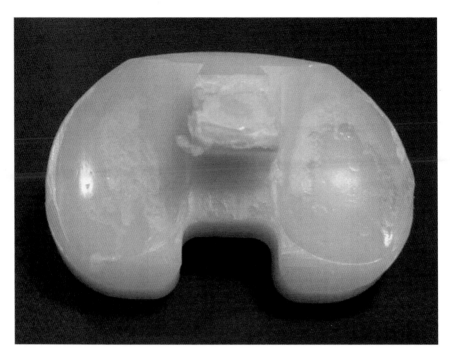

Fig. 6.43 Comparison of Post and Articular Surface Damage.

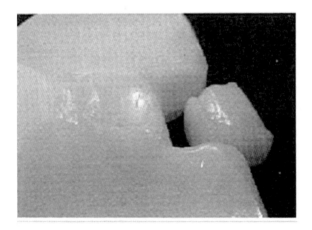

Fig. 6.44 Fractured NexGen Post – A Three Year Retrieval [54].

As may be seen from Fig. 6.44 catastrophic, fracture of the post may also be the result of the excessive stresses on the post characteristic of PS devices.

d) ***Discussion***

The cam-post stresses found in all the PS designs are grossly excessive. This is particularly true since axial rotation is expected in moderate and deep flexion where the post and cam are engaged under load will magnify these stresses in fixed bearing devices as a result of the edge contact produced. In all post and cam designs the contact stresses are well above the estimated compressive yield strength of UHMWPe. From an engineering viewpoint it is sufficient to know that such stresses will produce yielding and early fatigue. It means little if they are estimated to be two times or three times higher than the yield strength other than that such failure will occur more rapidly with higher stress. That stresses in a device are higher than yield is considered enough to disqualify such a device from human use by any reasonable engineering criteria. The retrieval specimens of Figures 6.40-6.44 demonstrate this as does the analysis of the retrievals of Refs. 87, 88. Thus, enhanced posterior stability is likely gained at the expense of greater wear as is shown by McEwen [89] who found, in knee simulator testing, that a typical, incongruent, fixed bearing as used in PS knee replacement wears at a rate four times higher than a semi-congruent design such as the LCS.

Newer designs have attempted to address the problem of excessive post against cam contact stress. Unfortunately although these designs are a significant improvement over those studied here they are, nevertheless, still highly over stressed as noted by Akasagi et al [56]. These calculations also ignore the magnifying effect of axial rotation.

Although excessive contact stresses is the most significant defect of such designs, patellar problems associated with patellofemoral track recession and added bone loss associated with cam to post PS fixed bearing knees are serious functional disadvantages. The use of such knees was probably justified in the past. The enhanced dislocation resistance provided by such designs solved the more serious problem of posterior dislocation encountered with earlier fixed bearing designs. The damage potential associated with increased wear is long-term in nature while dislocation is short term and catastrophic.

Whether the use of such devices is still justified is, however, questionable. Advances in knee replacement concepts, particularly the use of mobile bearings, have allowed the development of devices with improved stability against dislocation and subluxation. The congruity of mobile bearing knees, coupled with the use of posterior inclination of the tibial components substantially increases the engagement between the femoral and tibial components thus substantially increasing A/P stability. The thirty - year successful, clinical experience with the LCS and its derivatives shows that a cam - to – post element is not needed to adequately control posterior dislocation [75].

The key to dislocation stability, other than proper implant design, is reliable control of flexion tension and tibial component positioning and inclination. This is readily achieved by appropriate current, well-developed, surgical technique as shown in Ref. [90].

If A/P stability is not needed the question of whether to use PS cam to post elements reduces the risk to benefit associated with femoral roll back. The most widely used of the PS designs evaluated fails to provide any significant roll back and yet has the best lever arm properties. Of the rest most, unfortunately, provide little, if any, roll back for stair climbing where improved quadriceps function is quite important. A few provide significant roll back, such as, arising from a chair where there is 100° of flexion and for the Asian population where one sees about 130° of active flexion [1]. With regard to arising from a chair one would expect little functional benefit since both legs, as well as the arms, are usually used for this activity. With regard to flexion at 130° only two of the PS designs allow such flexion. However, only the LCS-PS allows the 20° of axial rotation needed to obtain such flexion [1]. Unfortunately, the LCS-PS knee studied here has been withdrawn due to patellofemoral problems.

The question, therefore, is whether the added risk and complexity of providing forced roll back is justified by the improved function generated by this roll back? Such improvement is difficult to show clinically [44] or even theoretically and thus this question is not readily answered. At this time, however, there seems little proven reason to use the available PS designs studied for their roll back properties.

Although the past use of PS knees to control posterior dislocation represented a major advance at the time they were first introduced, the advent of conforming, mobile bearings as well as advancements in surgical instrumentation and technique, seem to have also provided needed stability. Thus, one should consider whether the risk associated with problems identified in PS devices is justified since, as has been shown by a quarter century of clinical experience, adequate stability against posterior dislocation can be provided by improved surgical techniques and currently available designs, not using a post and cam.

6.5.2 Third Generation Designs

6.5.2.1 The Oxford Knee

The Oxford knee has demonstrated success as a medial compartment unicondylar replacement and has been approved by the U.S. FDA on the basis of a Pre Market Approval (PMA) application. It is contraindicated for lateral or bicompartmental replacement [91-93].

The Oxford design has design deficiencies that limit its use. The most important is the excessive translation of the lateral bearing resulting from a single radius of curvature femoral component to replace a condyle with a diminishing curvature posteriorly [94], as illustrated in Fig 6.45.

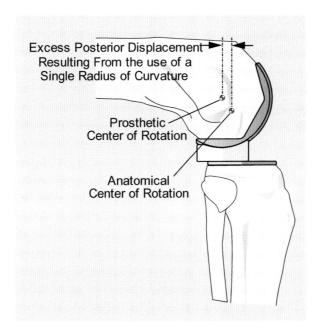

Fig. 6.45 Excessive Posterior Bearing Displacement Due to use of a Single Radius of Curvature of the Femoral Component.

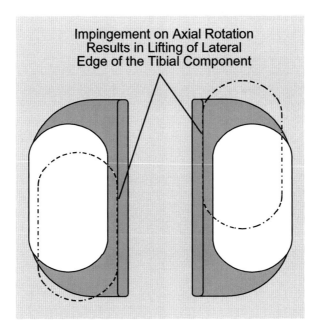

Fig. 6.46 Lack of Sufficient Axial Rotation Results in Tensile Stress at Fixation Interface.

In addition, lack of adequate axial rotation, as shown in Fig 6.46, and lack of a patellofemoral articulation limit its application as a bicruciate retaining device or a tricompartmental replacement.

6.5.2.2 The LCS

a) *Contact Stresses and Wear*
1) Tibiofemoral Articulation

A theoretical and experimental contact stress study in Section 2.4.5.2 of the LCS and other fixed bearing knees [95], demonstrates the superiority of the mobile bearing tibiofemoral articulation. It may be seen from this study that only the contact stresses in the area (mobile bearing) type are within reasonable limits. The other types (fixed bearings) have stresses, greatly exceeding acceptable limits, even approaching, or exceeding the compressive yield stress of UHMWPe. Furthermore, contact stress in the LCS is essentially unaffected by axial rotation while such rotation normally substantially increases contact stress in fixed bearing knees [96].

These results have been corroborated by the study of White et al [97]. That study found a mean contact stress at 750 lbs load and 15° flexion of about 2MPa for the LCS and about 13MPa for typical fixed bearing knees. Converting mean stress to peak stress and compensating for the different loads used in Ref. [97] yields an LCS stress of 3.8MPa and 25 MPa for typical fixed bearing knees. These values are in close agreement with those of Ref. [73].

2) Patellofemoral Articulation

A theoretical analysis of prosthetic patellofemoral contact stresses [98] demonstrates the situation that exists with regard to patellar prostheses today. This analysis studies the articulating geometry and excludes the effect of metal-backing. Metal-backed prostheses (except for the area contact type, where thickness does not affect stress) would have about double these calculated values. The articular geometries studied are shown in Fig. 6.47.

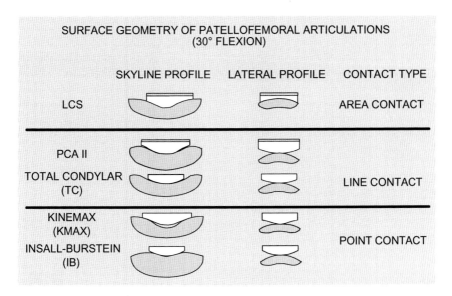

Fig. 6.47 Patellofemoral Geometries Studied.

The results are given in Fig. 6.48.

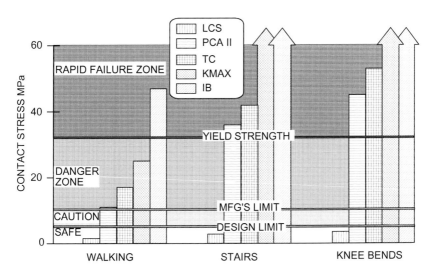

Fig. 6.48 Computed Contact Stress in Current Prosthetic Patellofemoral Articulations.

It may be seen that stresses in fixed bearing patellae are far beyond the abilities of UHMWPe [84]. The poor performance of such designs was readily predictable and has been thoroughly documented [8, 99-106].

3) Wear Simulator Testing

An early two million cycle simulator test of the Total Condylar and LCS Meniscal Bearing Knees test showed serious pitting of the Total Condylar developing within 100K cycles, and only minor abrasive wear of the mobile bearing knee at the end of the test [20]. Somewhat later a new simulator was used in an effort to obtain quantitative data on knee wear as described in Section 2.4.5.2. These tests confirmed the expected dramatic superiority with respect to wear of the LCS compared to all the tested fixed bearing devices.

4) Mobility

The stability study of Postac et al [107] demonstrates the mobility of the New Jersey LCS proving that the low contact stress of mobile bearing designs is matched by low constraint forces, as seen in Fig. 6.49.

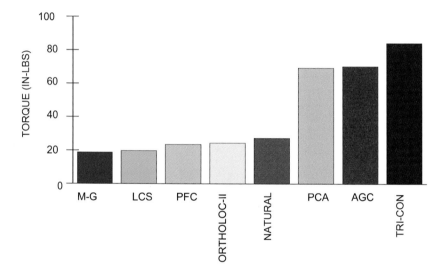

Fig. 6.49 Axial Torque at 5° Rotation with 430 lbs Axial Load.

5) Clinical Results

Long-term, multicenter clinical trials, involving thousands of patients, have demonstrated the safety and efficacy of the New Jersey LCS Knee Replacement System [70, 75]. The results from Refs. [108] and [109] are shown in Figs. 6.50 and 6.51 respectively.

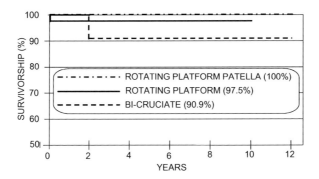

Fig. 6.50 Survivorship of New Jersey LCS Knees [108].

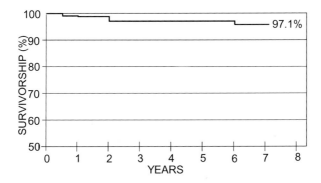

Fig. 6.51 Survivorship of 1140 New Jersey LCS Knees [109].

The long-term survival rate of the Bicruciate Retaining device was not satisfactory as may be seen from Fig. 6.50. Most of these failures were the result of meniscal bearing fracture as described in the next section. The Bicruciate Retaining device was initially well accepted but gradually declined in popularity due to its difficulty in implantation and the excellent performance of the Rotating Platform. Thus, its use was gradually phased out.

The long-term survival rate of the Unicompartmental device was also not satisfactory with a survival rate at 10 years of only about 85%. Nevertheless a version of this device is still marketed by DePuy Orthopaedics.

The clinical results for the LCS Rotating Platform have been, however, excellent. Note particularly the extremely low rate of patellar complications in Fig. 6.50. This is typical of clinical studies of the New Jersey LCS demonstrating that properly designed metal-backed patellae do work.

Conversely the survivorship of early fixed bearing knees was quite poor. Metal-backed fixed patellae were particularly poor. This poor performance is readily predictable on the basis of the theoretical and experimental analysis described earlier.

6) Fracture of Meniscal Bearings

This problem is of interest since it demonstrates that unexpected problems may arise. Furthermore, the analysis used to identify its cause and to develop a solution should be of interest to implant designers.

During the FDA clinical trial, which was initiated in 1980, six patients of one of the surgical centers involved in the trial experienced early fractures of meniscal bearings. These fractures occurred within three years after implantation. Such failure was limited to this center during the clinical trial. A preliminary investigation indicated that knee laxity appeared to be a factor in the failures. Defective polyethylene was also suspected. After the conclusion of the FDA trial, and after general sale of the LCS, additional fractures were documented. The problem persists today being most common in long-term implantations. The estimated failure rate for this mode of failure is about 1% in 10 years of use.

Since 1985 a total of 23 sets of retrieved meniscal bearings and the patient histories were studied. All but three sets were 10mm bearings. It was found that although knee laxity and malalignment was often present in such failures. This failure also occurred to a substantial degree in tight, well aligned, knees. One common feature was, however, present in this batch of fractured bearings. In all but two bearings, where the initiation points of the cracks could be determined, the crack initiated at the lateral edge of the articulating surface. In the two exceptions, the fracture initiated in the male dovetail of the bearing.

Consider first the problem of crack initiation at the lateral edge of the articular surface. Contact pressures will produce a force component which loads the edge of the bearing as shown in Fig. 6.52. Knee malalignment and laxity increase the value of this edge load.

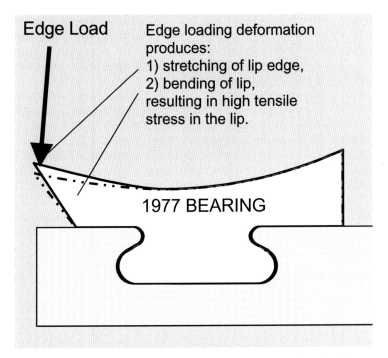

Fig. 6.52 Effect of edge loading on the lateral lip of a meniscal bearing.

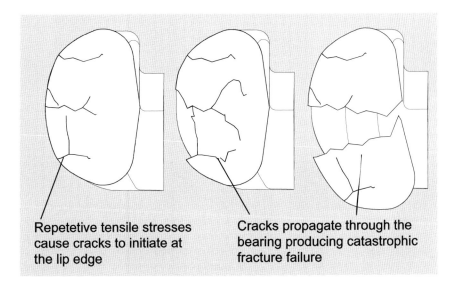

Fig. 6.53 Crack initiation, propagation, and coalescence producing catastrophic meniscal bearing failure.

Loading of the overhanging lip at the lateral bearing edge produces deformation of the lip which includes stretching and bending of the lip. Stretching results in a hoop stress, and therefore, tensile stresses in the lip edge. Bending produces additional tensile stresses at the superior surface of the lip. This qualitative evaluation was verified by a three dimensional finite element study of the effects produced by such loading.

These stresses, under repetitive loading conditions, can result in the development of cracks at the edge of the lateral bearing lip. Such cracks will then propagate through the bearing producing catastrophic failure as shown in Fig. 6.53.

The effect of bearing thickness in such fractures is important only in that thinner bearings have thinner, weaker lips. Compressive contact stresses are not a significant factor in these failures. No failures initiated by excessive compressive stress were observed.

No investigation into the nature of the UHMWPe used in these bearings was performed by Depuy. Collier, however, has investigated this issue [110]. His laboratory has examined 91 fractured, retrieved, meniscal bearings. Of these, 64 are made of polyethylene with significant internal fusion defects.

In summary, bearing fractures are the result of design, material defects, and knee malalignment and laxity.

The solution to the design problem was to eliminate the overhanging lip, as shown in Figs. 6.54 and 6.55.

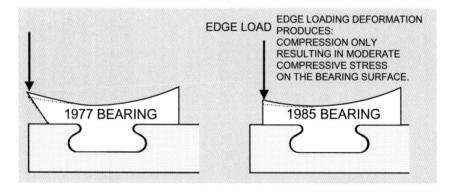

Fig. 6.54 Elimination of the overhanging lip - transverse view.

This design modification was introduced in 1989. At about the same time DePuy introduced Enduron a high quality, defect free, UHMWPe. These changes, along with improved intraoperative evaluation, have apparently eliminated these fracture problems. In the five years since the introduction of these changes no bearings of the new design have fractured. Since with the early bearings a significant, but small, number of fractures occurred when the use of the device was limited to clinical trials, the lack of fractures of the new bearings in wide spread general use, over a longer period of time than the trial, is strong evidence that the fracture problems were solved.

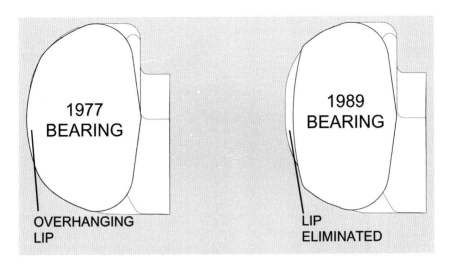

Fig. 6.55 Elimination of the overhanging lip - superior view.

6.5.2.3   PFC Sigma RPF

It is a sad truth but many, if not most, orthopaedic implants are designed for the desires, rather than the needs of the marketplace. In doing so scientific and engineering principles are often ignored or discarded. A case in point is the DePuy PFC Sigma RPF posterior stabilized total knee replacement.

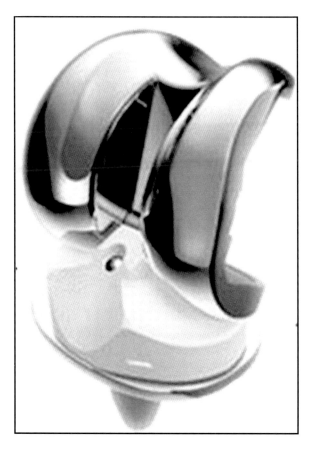

Fig. 6.56 PFC Sigma RPF Knee Replacement.

The PFC Sigma RPF is a derivative of the PFC Sigma RP which is itself a derivative of the fixed bearing PFC Sigma. The PFC Sigma RP was derived from the LCS Knee by adapting the LCS rotating platform and bearing to the PFC Sigma and modifying the articulating surfaces of the PFC Sigma so that they function similar to the LCS. This produced the PFC Sigma RP device with performance characteristics similar to those of the highly successful LCS.

The posterior stability concept had become very popular. This led DePuy into the development and introduction of a posterior stabilized LCS device. This device quickly failed and was withdrawn from the market. It was apparent that the roll back produced by PS devices is incompatible with the semi-congruent LCS articulating surfaces which do not allow much roll back.

When DePuy adapted the post and cam concept to the PFC Sigma RP they avoided the problem encountered with the LCS by using the incongruent, fixed bearing, tibiofemoral articulating surfaces of the original PFC Sigma. This action, in effect substituted the unneeded, scientifically unsound properties of the cam – to – post concept for the needed and sound properties of semi-congruent articulation. Thus, it substituted needed performance for market perception.

The study of Ref. [111] clearly shows this as is illustrated in Fig. 6.57 where the lighter shades indicate higher stress.

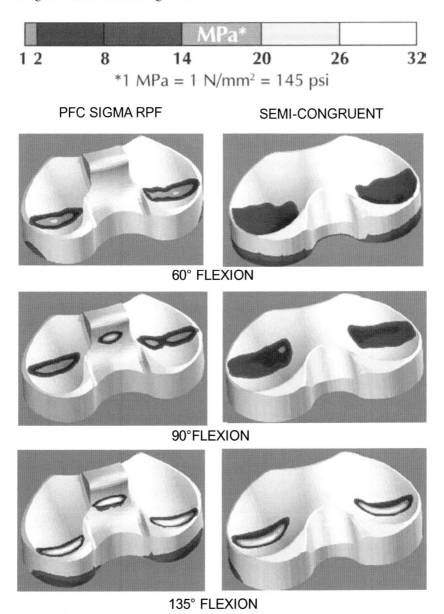

Fig. 6.57 Comparison of Stresses in the PFC Sigma RPF and a Semi-Congruent Bearing.

It may be seen that the stresses in the PFC Sigma RPF are substantially higher than in a semi-congruent design and that the stresses on the post contact area are significantly higher than on the articulating surface of the PFC Sigma RPF bearing.

6.6   Evolution of the B-P Knee System

The B-P knee replacement systems have evolved over the last 30 years. This evolutionary process provides important insights into the science and art of knee implant design.

6.6.1   Modified Total Condylar

In 1976 the New Jersey (B-P) Mark I knee was developed by Drs. Buechel and Pappas. This design is a variation of the original Total Condylar. The primary change was an improved patellar prosthesis and anterior femoral flange. The design improves on the patellar design of the Total Condylar, which was inadequately designed in this regard, by having a bump in the area where patellar compression loads are high. The improved congruety is illustrated in Figs. 6.58 and 6.59 where the right hand figures are those of the Total Condylar.

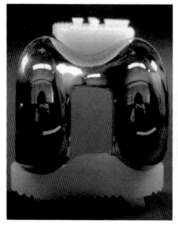
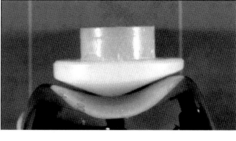

Fig. 6.58 Comparison of Profile Views of a NJ and Button Patellar Replacement.

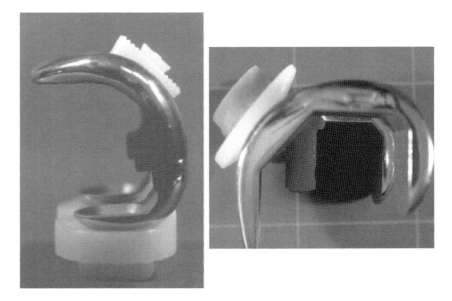

Fig. 6.59 Comparison of the Lateral of a NJ and Button Patellar Replacement.

6.6.2   The LCS

Experience with the Mark I knee, which was quite good, led directly to the development of the New Jersey, Mark II, Mobile Bearing Knee in 1977. Failure of the Mark I to flex beyond 90°, when the cruciates were retained, led to

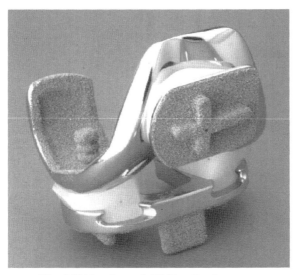

Fig. 6.60 New Jersey LCS Knee Replacement.

the conclusion that flatter tibial surfaces were needed to allow roll back. Unfortunately, analysis of the condylar geometry showed that the Total Condylar geometry was already over stressed and further flattening of the tibial surface was not allowable using any rational engineering basis. The mobile bearing concepts which had been previously used in the earlier Buechel – Pappas' shoulder and trunion-cylindrical ankle were adapted to produce the mobile bearing knee design in 1977. This device was licensed to DePuy in the late 1970's.

This knee system was approved by the FDA on the basis of a formal PMA and supporting clinical studies in 1985. DePuy has been selling various versions of this device since that time.

Drs. Buechel and Pappas worked with DePuy to develop the second generation of the LCS, the LCS "Complete", until their relationship with DePuy was severed in 2004. Since this termination, they developed a refined fifth generation NJ knee version, the Buechel-Pappas Mark V Knee Replacement System.

6.6.3   The B-P Mark V Knee System

The Buechel-Pappas Mark V System comprises a system of elements which can treat a wide variety of pathologies and surgeon preferences. The implants are available in six sizes with four bearing thicknesses for each size. A narrow femoral component, a partially conforming fixed bearing, a hinge and modular revision components are available.

6.6.3.1   Narrow Femoral Component

The recent introduction of a "gender specific" femoral component has raised the issue of the variation in the medial/lateral to anterior/posterior aspect ratio of the distal femur and other geometry variations. Although the aspect ratio of the average female knee is slightly less than the male knee this difference is small compared to the individual variations found in males as well as females [112]. This sexual dimorphism in the aspect ratio seems insufficient to justify a gender specific knee except, perhaps, for marketing reasons.

The differences in individual variation, however, are sufficient to justify a set of narrower femoral components for use in both male and female patients where the standard width femoral component is too wide for a particular patient. As a result the authors have developed "Narrow" femoral components, which are 7.6% narrower than the standard components, for such use.

Knee System Implant Availability, Sizing and Catalog Numbers

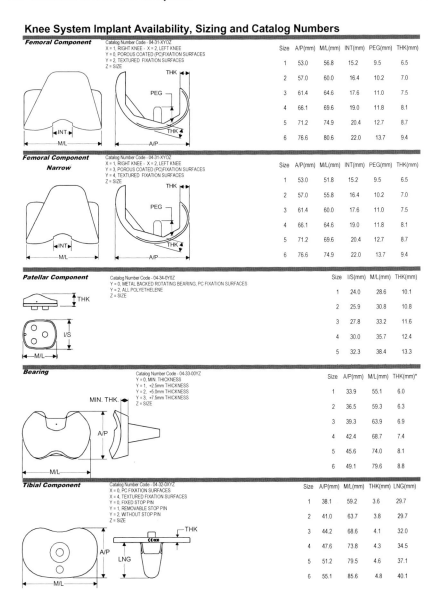

Fig. 6.61 Buechel-Pappas Knee Replacement System.

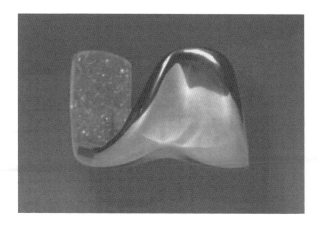

Fig. 6.62 Narrow B-P Femoral Component.

This Narrow, Femoral Component avoids such gender specific characteristics, such as a thinner femoral flange and lack of normal axial rotation of some of the competitive designs. The thinner femoral flange of some gender specific devices reduces the engagement of the patella with the femoral component increasing the risk of patellar subluxation. This is a problem much more common in females than in males and thus seems contradictory for female knees [113].

6.6.3.2 Partially Conforming Bearing

Notwithstanding the clear design deficiencies of typical fixed bearing knees and the thirty year successful use of mobile bearing knees, many surgeons, for reasons unfathomable to the authors, preferred to use fixed bearing knees in their patients. To satisfy such surgeons while minimizing the problem of articular surface overloading common to fixed bearing knees the authors developed a lower contact stress fixed bearing knee for use in less demanding patients.

The Buechel-Pappas (B-P) Partially Conforming Tibial Bearing is an asymmetric bearing which is perfectly congruent with the B-P Mark V Femoral Component on the medial condyle and in partially congruent line contact on the lateral condyle. In this regard it mimics the natural knee, which has much greater congruity, on its medial articulation.

The bearing allows ±20° of axial rotation around the medial condyle. Such rotation is sufficient for all normal activities including deep knee flexion associated with squatting [1]. This degree of rotation greatly exceeds that of typical knees, particularly the posterior stabilized types, which do not provide sufficient axial rotation for normal activities [2].

The allowable compressive stress under repeated loads is given in Ref. [84] as 10MPa. Values below this recommendation have only been achieved in mobile bearing knees [73]. These reported values, as well as all others assume shared, equal loading of the condyles.

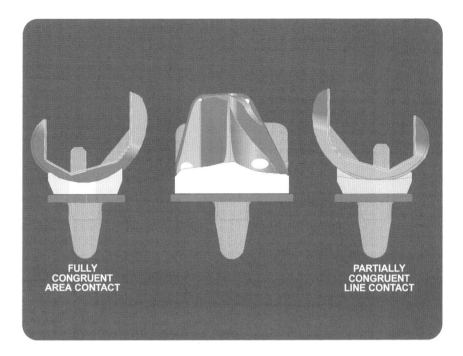

Fig. 6.63 Partially Conforming B-P Bearing.

The actual stress is actually substantially higher since during peak loading most of the load is taken by the medial condyle.

In the B-P Mark V Conforming and Partially Conforming Bearings the contact stress on the medial condyle during peak loading, using the higher load of the medial condyle, is about 3 MPa. This is well below the 10MPa recommendation and a "safe" stress of 5MPa.

On the lateral side forces are not well understood except that they are relatively low in normal gait. Pathological gait is usually quite different. As a conservative estimate it will be taken as one half the peak load. Under this assumption the contact stress on the lateral condyle of the B-P partially conforming knee is about 8MPa, which is less than the recommended limit but higher than the safe limit. These calculations are based on expected loads in a perfectly aligned knee. Misalignment can have a major impact on contact stresses in the knee.

This latter value is several times higher than in the Conforming Bearing. Thus, the Partially Conforming Bearing is intended for less demanding patients than those for whom the Conforming Bearing is best used.

The value of the contact stress in the lateral condyle of the Partially Conforming Bearing is, however, a fraction of the values found in typical incongruent bearings. Thus, the Partially Conforming Bearing is more resistant to wear and other effects of load and motion than typical fixed bearing knees.

6.6.3.3 Revision Components

The B-P Mark V Knee modular revision components are used with stem extensions to provide additional stability where there is insufficient bone stock or other deficiency as shown in Fig. 6.4.

The stem connection is reliable, easy to use and clinically proven in more than a decade of use in B-P modular hip stem components. It avoids the potential for loosening and micro motion present in typical taper stem connections and the associated problems of micro motion and metallic wear debris by a connection that avoids micromotion.

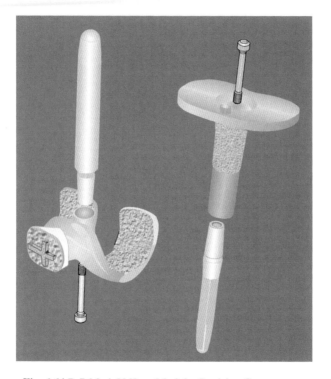

Fig. 6.64 B-P Mark V Knee Modular Revision Components.

6.6.3.4 B-P Hinge Knee

Primary load bearing of the B-P Mark II Hinge Knee is carried by the tibiofemoral articulating surfaces and not by the hinge element as it is in other hinge knee designs. This allows for the use of a relatively small hinge which needs only to resist shear forces and not the much greater compression forces. The tibiofemoral articulating surfaces of this knee are fully congruent in all phases of flexion resulting in very low contact stress for all activities.

The use of a small hinge reduces the necessary bone resection to less than that associated with most Posterior Stabilized designs as shown in Fig. 6.65.

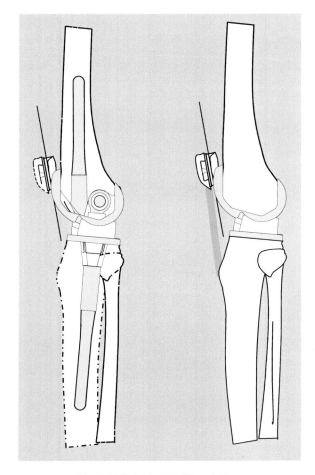

Fig. 6.65 B-P Mark II Hinged Knee.

6.6.3.5 Backside Wear

The B-P Mark V Tibial Platform surfaces contacting the bearing are all highly polished ceramic. As a result "backside" wear commonly observed in retrieved bearings [114] is greatly reduced.

6.6.4 Design of the LCS, Mark II, Knee Replacement

The LCS and its variants are a highly successful knee replacement used worldwide for more than a quarter century. The design rationale for such knee replacements needs to be understood. It can provide a basis for successful design of future knee replacement systems.

6.6.4.1 Tibial Components

a) Metallic Tray Reinforcement

The use of a metal platform, which is required with mobile bearings, is highly desirable in itself even when used with fixed bearing elements. Metallic platforms minimize interface tension and maximize uniformity of interface compression as illustrated in Fig. 6.66. Mobile bearings simply make optimal use of the metal platform by allowing the bearing elements to move providing joint mobility without introducing unnecessary bearing incongruity.

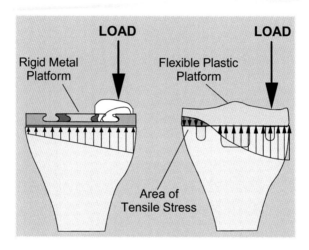

Fig. 6.66 Reinforcing Effect of Metal Platform.

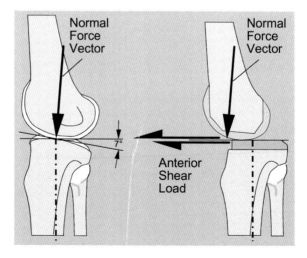

Fig. 6.67 Added Joint Forces Resulting from Perpendicular Tibial Platform Placement.

b) Effects of Tibial Plane Inclination

If the tibial component is placed perpendicular to the tibial axis, as is the norm, shearing forces are introduced at the articulating surfaces and prosthetic interfaces as seen in Fig. 6.67.

Further, since with a perpendicular tibial bearing surface the normal ligament pattern is not duplicated, flexion must be accompanied by stretching of the ligaments as illustrated in Fig. 6.68.

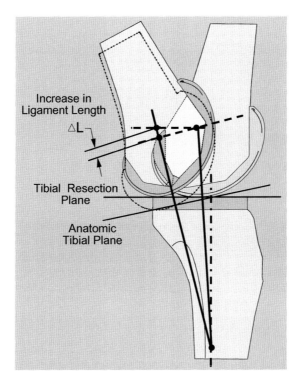

Fig. 6.68 Stretching of Ligaments on Flexion due to Perpendicular Tibial Placement.

This results in loss of flexion and added posterior compression force producing anterior lift (and tension). This action increases the joint reaction force, and reduces compression uniformity. The lack of posterior tibial inclination is probably responsible for flexion problems with the PCA and is likely the reason the designers of the PCA used an anterior screw in an attempt to avoid anterior lift.

A compromise solution is used in the "Insall-Burstein" Knee which uses a perpendicular resection but a wedge type tibial component producing a posteriorly inclined prosthetic plane as illustrated in Fig. 6.69.

This approach eliminates shear at the articular surface providing a partial solution. Unnecessary shear at the bone-prosthesis interface remains, however. It should also be noted that a perpendicular resection requires additional anterior tibial resection compared to an inclined cut as seen in Fig. 6.70.

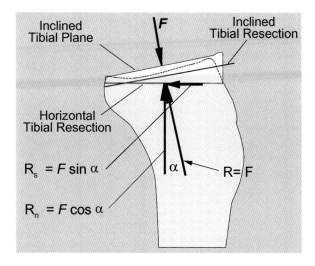

Fig. 6.69 Interface Shear Resulting from a Perpendicular Resection.

Further, since the tibial plane is not parallel to the distal femoral resection, an anterior-posterior variation in the position of the femur relative to the tibia will produce a variation in prosthetic gap since the path of the femur is along the inclined plane and is not parallel to the distal femoral resection. Thus inclining the articular surface, but not the tibial resection, provides only a partial solution to the problems of a perpendicular tibial cut.

On the other hand, a posteriorly inclined tibial and femoral resection used with LCS meniscal bearing tibial components, results in the elimination of A-P interfacial shear and a consistent prosthetic gap as shown in Fig. 6.71.

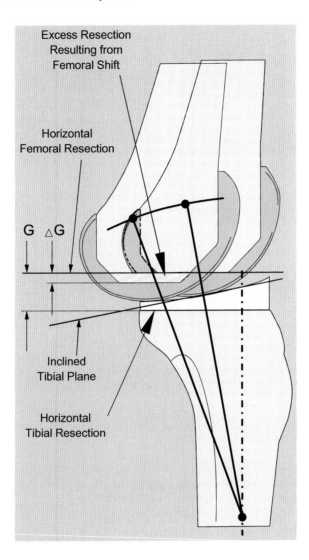

Fig. 6.70 Change in Femoral Position Produces a Change in Prosthetic Gap.

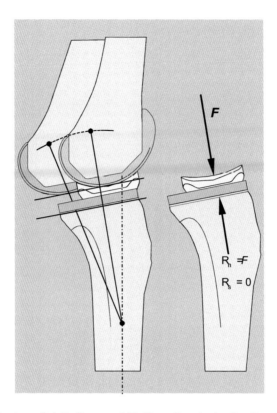

Fig. 6.71 Elimination of A-P Shear and Uniform Prosthetic Gap Results from Use of Inclined Femoral and Tibial Resections.

There is, however, a significant disadvantage associated with a posteriorly inclined cut. The cutting jig must be properly axially oriented with regard to the axis of the tibia or varus or valgus error will be introduced.

c) Rotating Tibial Platform
The function of the conical peg is to resist tipping due to off center tibial loading as illustrated in Fig. 6.73.

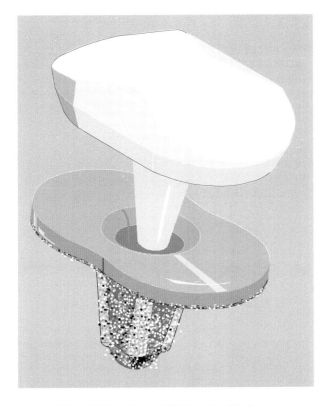

Fig. 6.72 New Jersey LCS Rotating Platform.

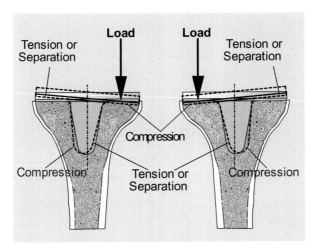

Fig. 6.73 Elastic Bed Effect on Tibial Component Due to Alternating Load.

Since the entire distal stem tip typically sees alternating tension and compression, ingrowth or long-term cement fixation is not expected at the tip. Thus, stress protection of the proximal tibia does not result from the fully porous coated stem. Rather the coating allows ingrowth of fibrous tissue that is felt to provide some degrees of tension load resistance and protection against pressure necrosis. When used with cement the coating prevents cement delamination from the metal and thus reduces the possibility of associated cement wear debris and bone lysis.

A conical peg is chosen for several reasons. These are:

1. Simplified preparation of the bone receiving the peg.
2. Ability to easily adjust the axial and transitional position of the tibial component as illustrated in Fig. 6.74.

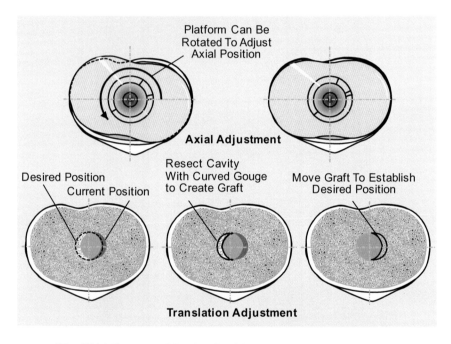

Fig. 6.74 Adjustment of Cruciate Sacrificing Tibial Component Position.

3. The ability to easily achieve a press fit, important in cementless use.
4. Provides a region for an effective load and wear resistant bearing connection.
5. Bone loss is limited to the central tibia where there is little bone of load carrying quality, and thus bone loss is not of great importance. Loss of bone in the condylar regions of the tibia associated with the fixation stem, where bone loss is of great importance is completely avoided.
6. Stress concentrations in the load bearing subchondral region associated with the sharp edges of the fins used in crossed fin stems are avoided.

The principal advantage of a crossed fin or rectangular stem to improve torsional resistance is not important in this design since the rotating platform is free of axial constraints and therefore does not exert significant torque on the interface. Thus, for this application, a conical stem is superior to a crossed fin stem.

Where both cruciates are absent, lack of sufficient anterior-posterior soft tissue restraints, requires that A-P stability be provided by the interaction of the bearing and the femoral component. The forces associated with these constraints must be supported by the interfaces between the bearing and the tibial platform. The Rotating Platform Bearing is, thus, designed to provide adequate shear resistance against fracture and wear at the bearing-platform connection.

d) Posterior Cruciate Tibial Platform

This design was intended for situations where only a viable posterior cruciate is available.

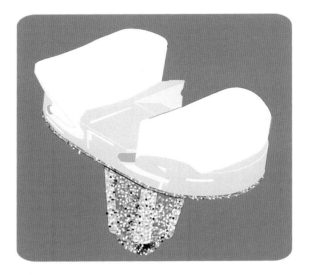

Fig. 6.75 Posterior Cruciate Retaining Platform.

This device, first introduced in 1984, utilizes the platform configuration of the Bicruciate Retaining Tibial Component with the fixation stem of the Cruciate Sacrificing Tibial Component. This is done to provide maximal system element compatibility. Thus, this device uses the same Meniscal Bearings as the Bicruciate device and similar instrumentation and surgical techniques as the cruciate sacrificing form. Since this design is easier to implant reliably than the Bicruciate retaining device form, some surgeons used the posterior cruciate retaining form even when a viable anterior cruciate is present by sacrificing the anterior cruciate.

This device was later replaced by an A/P gliding, robust, unit bearing replacing the dual meniscal bearing of the earlier device as illustrated in Fig. 6.76.

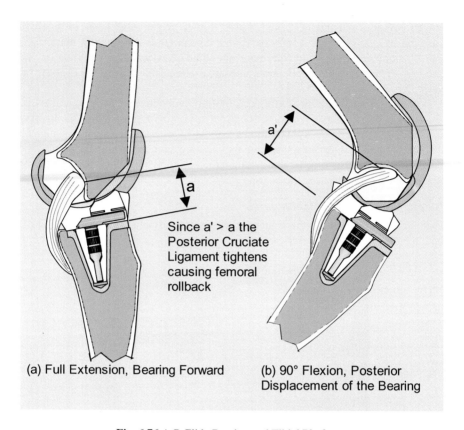

Since a' > a the
Posterior Cruciate
Ligament tightens
causing femoral
rollback

(a) Full Extension, Bearing Forward

(b) 90° Flexion, Posterior
Displacement of the Bearing

Fig. 6.76 A-P Glide Bearing and Tibial Platform.

The use of this device was, however, limited to use outside of the United States since it was not approved by the FDA.

Further, due to simplicity of surgical instrumentation, concerns for continued viability of the cruciates, and due to the inherent stability of the rotating platform device, some surgeons chose to routinely sacrifice the cruciates and implant the Cruciate Sacrificing Tibial Component in their entire patient population. Although there are now long-term clinical trials involving thousands of patients, the clinical justification for retaining or sacrificing, viable cruciate ligaments is not clearly established. As a result the cruciate sparing devices were abandoned.

6.6.4.2 Femoral Component

a) Sizing

In 1977, when the New Jersey LCS Knee System was developed, it was designed to use two sizes, The Standard and the Large. This was done in order to minimize inventory associated with the system. Size of inventory was then important since the amount of inventory, even with only two sizes, was greater than other knee designs which, at the time, did not use a systems approach. A typical knee of the time had only one type of UHMWPe tibial component rather than the variety available with the LCS system.

Published data [115] was used to select a width of 65mm for the Standard femoral component and 75mm for the large as shown in Fig. 6.78.

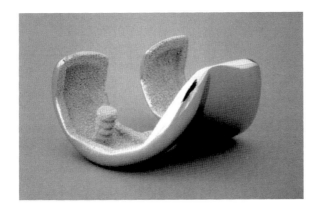

Fig. 6.77 New Jersey LCS Femoral Component.

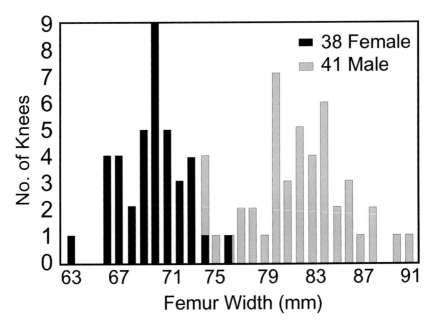

Fig. 6.78 Distribution of Femur Widths [115].

The tibial components, of a given size, were made the same width as the femoral components, of the same size, although the tibial component should be slightly wider to provide, on average, the best tibial coverage. The tibial component was made smaller to prevent tibial component overhang where, the best fit femoral component is slightly large for the patient, significant amount of tibia is resected, or the tibia is relatively small compared to the femur.

When the additional Standard plus and Large Plus components were introduced in about 1985 the original tibial sizes were retained since many distributors did not want the additional sizes. This produced a situation, which when four sizes are employed, the best tibial size for the closest femoral size match is typically the next highest size tibial component. Thus, for a patient where a Standard femoral component provides the best fit on the femur a Standard Plus tibial component usually provides the best fit onto the tibia.

b) Distal Femoral Resection

The only change made to the femoral component since 1977 was a change to a 15° distal fixation surface. This change was made in 1978.

Originally a "femur first approach" was employed as shown in Fig. 6.79.

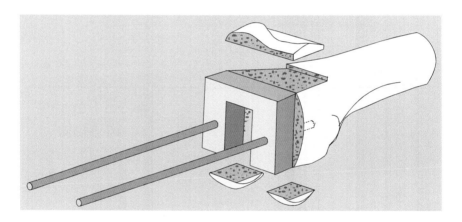

Fig. 6.79 Original Femur First Approach Instrumentation in 1977.

This approach, unfortunately, produced both a variable extension gap and a variable flexion gap which could not be controlled by careful surgery. An attempt to control the flexion gap lead to the abandonment of the femur first approach in 1978 and the adaptation of Insall's "tibia first" approach.

This new approach, although improving the situation did not entirely solve the problem. The remaining problem was discussed earlier. The distal femoral cut was not parallel to the anatomical tibial plane and thus, the prosthetic gap varied with femoral position.

Furthermore, since the femoral and distal resections are not parallel at full extension a spacer block cannot be used to check extension gap as illustrated in Fig. 6.80.

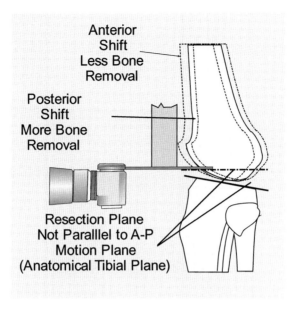

Fig. 6.80 Variable Resection Level Resulting From Variation in Femoral Position when a Perpendicular Femoral Resection is Used.

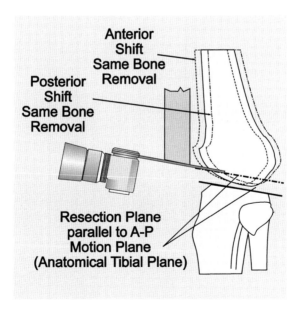

Fig. 6.81 Resection Level Independent of Femoral Position where an Inclined Distal Femoral Resection is Used.

When a properly inclined distal femoral resection is used variation in femoral position does not significantly affect the resection level, and since the femoral and tibial resections are parallel at full extension a spacer block can be used to check extension tension as is illustrated in Fig. 6.81.

Thus a 15° distal femoral cut is now used with the New Jersey LCS Femoral Component. The natural bow of the femur provides about 5° of flexion. This amount added to the 10° posterior inclination, relative to the anterior spine of the tibia, of the tibial component results in the need for a 15° femoral fixation surface. Properly aligned femoral and tibial components with the leg in full extension should appear as shown in Fig. 6.82.

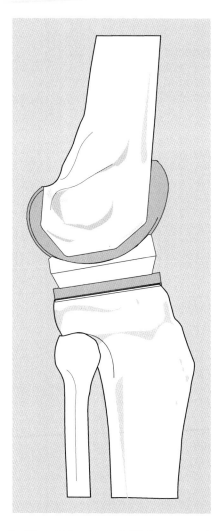

Fig. 6.82 Properly Aligned New Jersey LCS Components in Full Extension.

c) *Articular Surface*

The New Jersey LCS uses a common generating curve to form the articular surface of the femur as shown in Fig. 6.83.

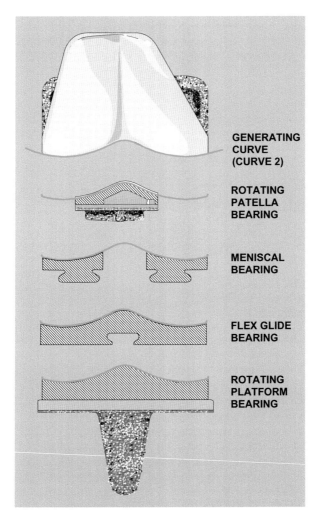

GENERATING
CURVE
(CURVE 2)

ROTATING
PATELLA
BEARING

MENISCAL
BEARING

FLEX GLIDE
BEARING

ROTATING
PLATFORM
BEARING

Fig. 6.83 Common Generating Curve.

The generating curve used for the femoral component is slightly different than the curve used to form the tibial and patellar articulating surfaces insuring that at least quasi-line contact will be maintained for all motion phases.

The generating curve used for the femoral component is 0.13% smaller than that used for the bearing surfaces. This difference was used to accommodate the curved tracks of the meniscal bearing tibial trays. Since on roll back it would be desirable to have the tracks produce posterior translation of the meniscal bearings the tracks would be straight. On axial rotation, however, the bearings should rotate with the femoral component.

In order to accommodate both motions curved tracks, with their centers of curvature on a vertical axis through of the spherical segment of the femoral components, are used. This accommodates axial rotation quite well. Some incongruity and M-L play is, however, introduced in order to accommodate roll back.

This generating curve is swept around a series of parallel axes to form the femoral articular shape.

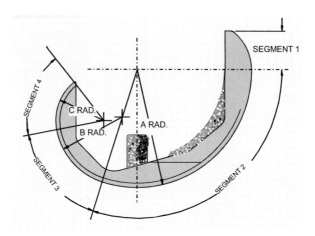

Fig. 6.84 Articulating Surface Segments of the Femoral Component.

Segment 2 the "Principal Load Bearing Segment" is generated by rotating the generating curve about an axis through the centers of the two main radii of Fig. 6.83. This produces two spherical regions in the Principal Load Bearing Segment. The tibial bearings have similar complimentary spherical surfaces, and thus all articulation in this region has quasi-congruent area contact. This produces near congruent tibiofemoral contact during peak load phases of walking and congruent patellar articulation during all motion phases except near full extension where patellofemoral compressive loads are very small.

Beyond around 35° of flexion the tibiofemoral articulation was typified by quasi-line contact. A reduced posterior radius of curvature for the femoral condyles is needed to provide anatomical motion without bearing extrusion.

This spherical surface also allows varus-valgus motion (Fig. 6.85).

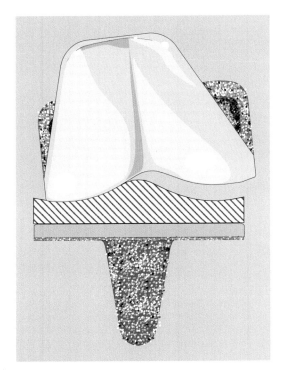

Fig. 6.85 Varus-Valgus Tilt without Loss of Congruent Contact.

and patellar tilt (Fig. 6.86) without loss of quasi-congruent contact.

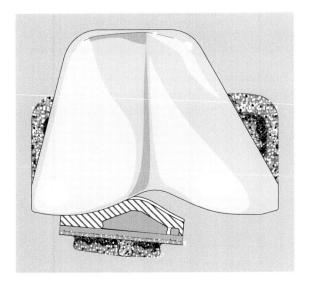

Fig. 6.86 Patellar Tilt Without Loss of Congruent Contact.

The use of a decreased posterior radius and posterior inclination of the tibial component significantly increases maximum potential flexion as shown in Fig. 6.87.

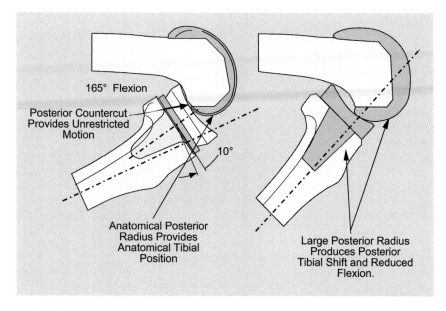

Fig. 6.87 Added Flexion Resulting from Smaller Posterior Femoral Condylar Radius.

This is a compromise also occurring in the natural knee. The designers of the Oxford Knee failed to make this compromise resulting in excessive lateral meniscal bearing dislocation. This issue is discussed in detail in Ref. [94].

The generating curve is designed to provide substantial medial-lateral stability where the tibial spine naturally providing this stability is resected as shown in Fig. 6.88.

In the case of the cruciate sacrificing device, needed anterior-posterior stability between the femur and bearing is provided by the congruency of the articulating surfaces and the posterior inclination of the tibial component as shown in Fig. 6.89.

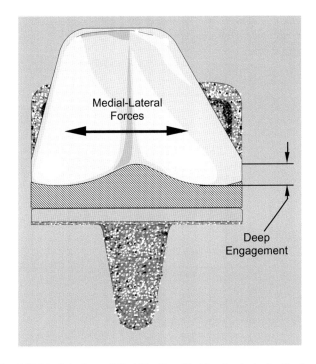

Fig. 6.88 Medial - Lateral Stability Provided by the Articular Surfaces.

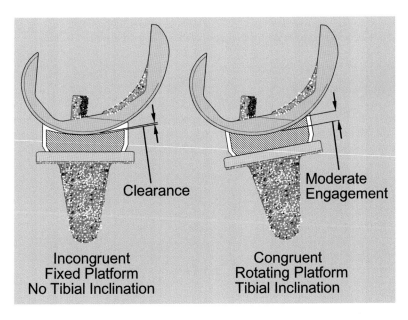

Fig. 6.89 Improved Anterior-Posterior Stability Resulting from Congruity and Posterior Tibial Component Inclination.

Additional A-P stability is provided by the "Deep-Dish" bearing, first introduced in 1986 and later adapted as part of the LCS Complete System as illustrated in Fig. 6.90.

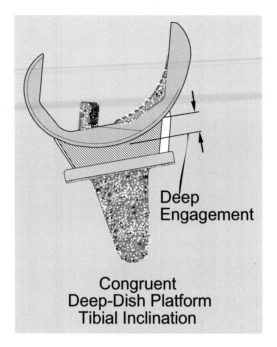

Fig. 6.90 Improved A-P Stability Available with the Deep-Dish Bearing.

d) Provision for Adequate Axial Rotation

It is a simple matter to produce a fully congruent design. Congruency, by itself, is, unfortunately, not sufficient. This is evidenced by the early Geomedic-Geometric designs which fail to provide adequate provision for axial rotation or femoral rollback. Mobility is needed along with congruity. Many later, incongruent, designs also fail to provide adequate axial rotation. Consider a typical incongruent design.

It may be seen that axial rotation can substantially change the nature of the surface contact as seen in Fig. 6.91. This is shown by McNamara et al in Ref. [96]. They also show in their study of the LCS that in properly designed mobile bearings the nature of the contact does not change since the bearing moves with the femoral component.

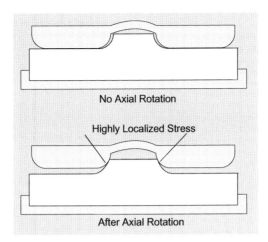

Fig. 6.91 Increased Contact Stress During Axial Rotation.

e) Provision for Abduction

Abduction of the knee occurs during the loading and swing phase of the walking cycle, and during other normal activities. Although loads during the swing phase are relatively low they are still significant. To minimize wear the articulating surfaces must accommodate such motion. The PCA design as well as the Miller-Gallante knee, Natural knee and the Osteonics knee are classic cases of failure to accommodate such motion since they use flat on flat articulating surfaces.

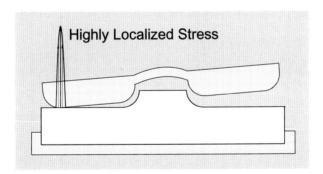

Fig. 6.92 Edge Loading During Abduction in Flat on Flat Design.

For such designs even low loads can produce large stresses under abduction as shown in Fig. 6.92. Use of properly designed femoral articulating surfaces (preferably spherical) can, however, properly accommodate abduction.

f) Femoral Roll Back

Similarly femoral roll back must be properly accommodated when the posterior cruciate is functional to minimize wear. This is best accomplished by use of mobile bearings, a femoral component with a decreasing posterior radius of curvature and use of a posterior tibial tilt as illustrated in Fig. 6.93.

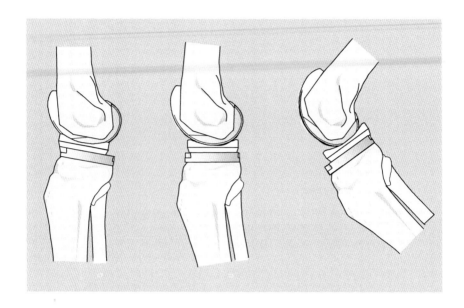

Fig. 6.93 Roll Back Accommodated by Meniscal Bearing Motion.

6.6.4.3 Patellar Component

Based on the principle that one should follow nature to the extent practical the prosthetic femoral sulcus should be anatomical, and should accommodate the natural lateral patellar tilt during flexion. This is achieved with the LCS. A natural femoral component sulcus cross sectional shape with a normal sulcus angle and a conforming patella are used as shown in Fig. 6.94.

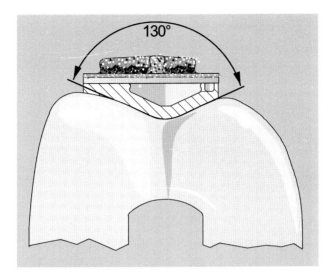

Fig. 6.94 Anatomic Prosthetic Articulation.

The spherical shape of the femoral condyles together with the lateral and middle patellar facets provide for patellar tilt without loss of congruency.

The patellar articulating surface likewise is anatomic, containing all but the odd facet as shown in Fig. 6.95.

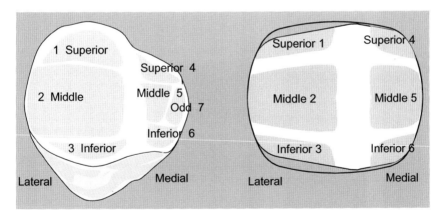

Fig. 6.95 Patella Facets.

A rotating patellar bearing is used to accommodate the normal axial patellar rotation.

One must, however, deviate from nature with regard to the femoral shape as viewed laterally in order to obtain congruity for both the patellofemoral and tibiofemoral articulations.

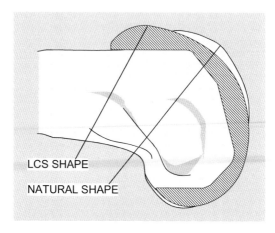

Fig. 6.96 Difference in Shape between the Femur and the LCS Femoral Component.

It is very difficult to attempt to reproduce the exact natural lateral sulcus shape. In particular the replication of the region between the femoral surface that articulates with both the patella, and with the tibia is hard to replicate.

In deep flexion the patella may articulate with the region of the femoral surface that articulates with the tibia near full extension. To accommodate this articulation overlap the LCS femoral component uses a common generating curve for the patellar and tibial articulations and a common radius of curvature for most of the patellar articulation, and part of the tibial articulation as shown in Figs. 6.96 and 6.97.

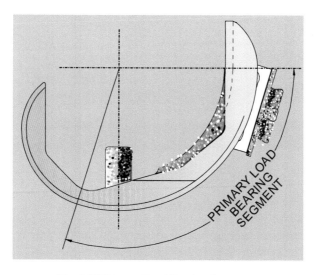

Fig. 6.97 Primary Load Bearing Segments.

This arrangement provides congruent contact throughout the patellofemoral motion range, except (mimicking the natural joint) near full extension where compressive loads are very low as shown in Fig. 6.98.

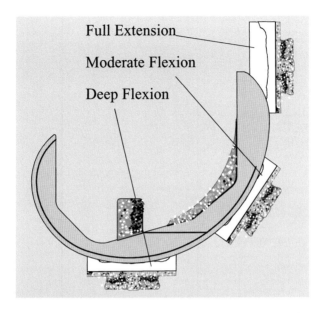

Fig. 6.98 Prosthetic Patellofemoral Contact.

Furthermore, the LCS femoral component design allows retention of the natural patella in many cases [116, 117]. Since the sulcus of the femoral component is anatomic in cross section, and since the natural patella always articulates against the same surface shape (except near full extension), the natural patella can more easily remodel to this constant, natural, shape than to the non-anatomical, varying shapes common to most other designs.

Metal-backing is not the problem. The problem is poor design. Metal-backing simply makes poor design worse. The solution is to follow nature (but not slavishly), follow basic engineering design principles, and to use some innovation. A rotating bearing, metal-backed design has been developed and found successful [108]. Other successful designs are possible if these principles above are observed.

6.6.5 The B-P Mark V Knee Replacement

6.6.5.1 Differences with the Mark I (LCS)

a) Femoral Component

The current Buechel-Pappas Femoral Component is an advanced fifth generation NJ device. It differs from the second generation device in five significant ways as shown in Figs. 6.99 and 6.100.

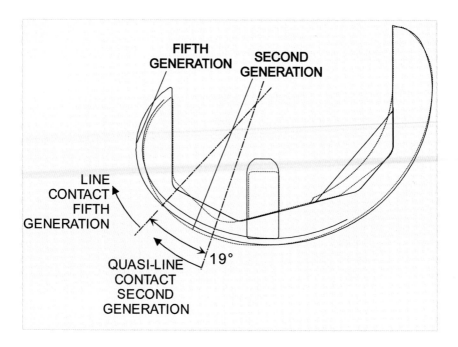

Fig. 6.99 Differences in the Lateral Shape of the second and Fifth Generation B-P (NJ) Femoral Components.

1. The primary load bearing segment arc is greater by 19° increasing the degree of congruent contact during flexion.
2. The minor incongruity needed to accommodate the meniscal bearings of the second generation is eliminated increasing congruity and reducing contact stress by 50%.
3. The distal and proximal condylar thicknesses are the same so that the prosthetic gaps can be precisely reproduced. The LCS posterior condylar thickness is about 1.5mm smaller than the distal thickness.
4. The fixation side of the sulcus is flat rather than curved as in the LCS providing contact with bone, rather than clearance in this region.
5. The medial anterior flange side wall angle is greater and the flange narrower eliminating the overhang often found in the B-P Mark II (NJ) Knee in this region.

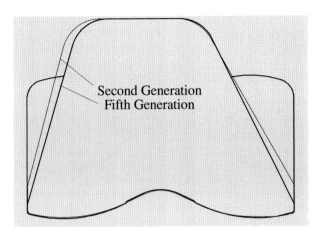

Fig. 6.100 Difference in the Frontal Shape of the Second and Fifth Generation B-P (NJ) Femoral Components.

b) Tibiofemoral Contact stresses

At flexion less than 30° the Mark I femoral component is actually in quasi-congruent, rather than fully congruent contact. Beyond 30° the contact changes to quasi-line contact. After about 90° the line contact becomes still more incongruent, further increasing stress.

Rather than the quasi-congruent or quasi-line contact articulating surfaces of the LCS the bearing articular surface in the B-P Mark V Tibial Bearing now conforms exactly to shape of the Femoral Component in the primary load bearing segment and in fully line contact elsewhere. This results in reduced contact stress in all motion and loading phases.

In addition the fifth generation device has an increased range of segment 2 contact. It is in fully congruent area contact until about 50° of flexion. Beyond that it remains in full line contact to its maximum flexion. A comparison of the contact in flexion is illustrated in Fig. 6.101.

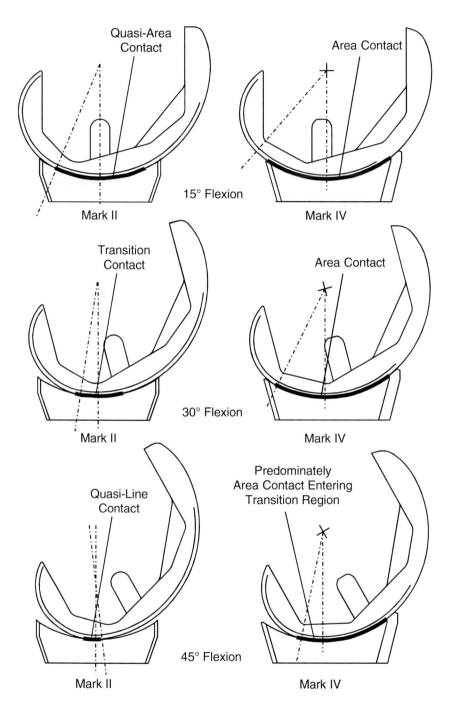

Fig. 6.101 Contact in the Mark III and Mark V Articulations.

A comparison of contact stresses for such articulations for the effects of greater congruity and greater congruent flexion range is given in Fig. 6.102 [118].

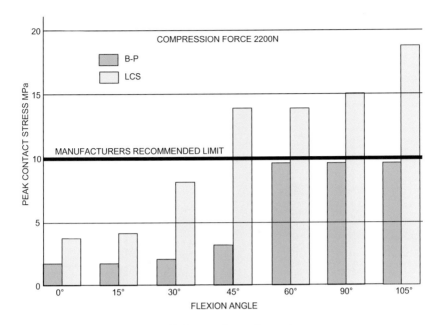

Fig. 6.102 Contact Stress Comparison.

It may be seen that stresses in the B-P are substantially lower than the LCS at all flexion angles.

c) Tibial Components

The B-P Tibial Platform (Fig. 6.103) is quite similar to the latest LCS version and is anatomically shaped. It differs from the LCS in that it contains a "Stop Pin" on its superior surface. This pin engages a slot or hole in the inferior surface of the Bearing to limit bearing rotation to prescribed limits.

Rotational dislocation of the rotating platform in the New Jersey LCS rotating platform knee is a significant complication (1.2% in the two PMA clinical trials). By proper attention to the maintenance of collateral ligament tension during implantation the rate of such dislocation can be kept acceptably low. Nevertheless, due to the absence of the cruciate ligaments, the principal anterior-posterior (A-P) and medial-lateral (M-L) stabilizers of the knee, the potential for such dislocation remains.

This instability characteristic is illustrated in Fig. 6.104. Due to the combined effects of an A-P shearing load, distraction of one of the condylar compartments, and a lax collateral ligament associated with the distracted compartment, the rotating bearing can be forced to rotate to a dislocated position. Only ligament tension sufficient to prevent the femoral condyle on the distracted side from climbing over the lip of the bearing can prevent such dislocation.

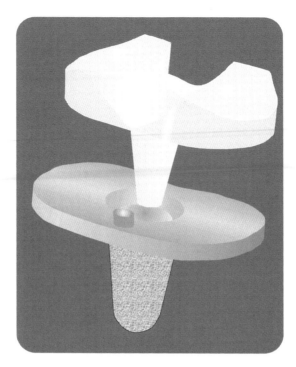

Fig. 6.103 B-P Tibial Platform.

Both A-P and M-L shift of the femur relative to the tibia as illustrated in Figs. 6.104(e) and (f) must accompany such dislocation. This action is called "spinout". The shearing force and the effect of the vertical rotation axis of the bearing accentuate such spinout. This type of subluxation cannot be reduced closed.

The spinout problem is solved by a rotational stop. The controlling concept, in providing a successful anti-spinout stop that will not adversely affect function, is to provide enough rotatory motion for all needed functions. Such motion should be limited so that if distraction allows disengagement and partial spinout, reapplying compressive force to the distracted condyle will produce self-reduction of the bearing.

The limit on axial rotation is produced by a Stop Pin on the tibial platform acting against the ends of a slot in the inferior surface of the bearing. These limits are not encountered during any activity but are reached only in the event of subluxation of the bearing from the femoral component.

Figs. 6.104(c) and (d) show a distracted femoral condyle on the bearing lip. In this position the anterior lip of the bearing is anterior to the center of the femoral condyle. If the bearing cannot rotate further so as to sublux as in Figs. 6.104(e) and (f) then when a compressive load is applied to the distracted condyle this side of the bearing will be forced anteriorly until the bearing has been returned into its normal position as shown in Figs. 6.104(a) and (b).

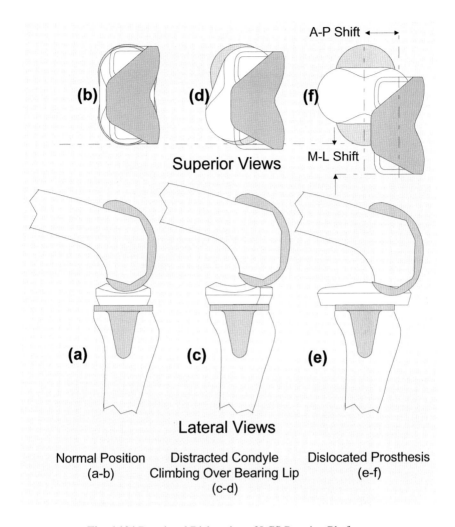

A-P Shift

(b)   **(d)**   **(f)**

Superior Views   M-L Shift

(a)   **(c)**   **(e)**

Lateral Views

Normal Position   Distracted Condyle   Dislocated Prosthesis
(a-b)   Climbing Over Bearing Lip   (e-f)
(c-d)

Fig. 6.104 Rotational Dislocation of LCS Rotating Platform.

The self-reducing feature of the tibial stop was first applied to the stop used in the patellar component of the LCS. The B-P Mark V knee provides ±45° axial rotation as shown in Fig. 6.105.

d)   Materials

The B-P Knee metallic components are made of TiN ceramic coated titanium alloy, a combination that is superior to Co-Cr alloy. Titanium is less expensive, stronger and more biocompatible. The ceramic coating is harder, more wear resistant and may greatly reduce polyethylene wear [119].

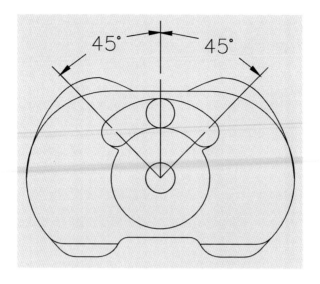

Fig. 6.105 Axial Rotation Limits.

The bearings are made of wear resistant 1050 UHMWPe sterilized by ethylene oxide.

e)   *Clinical Comparison*
The latest B-P knee clinical results appear to be a significant improvement over the original LCS as shown in Table 6.3.

Table 6.3 Comparison of LCS and B-P Posterior Cruciate Sacrificing Knees.

	153 LCS TKR's [120] 2-18yr (mean 9.5yr) (Gamma-in-Air Sterilization)	259 B-P TKR's [118] 2-18yr (mean 6.9yr) (Ethylene Oxide Sterilization)
Knee Score (NJOH)	87% Excellent	92% Excellent
Avg Range of Motion	0-107°	0-116°
Patient Satisfaction	94%	97%
Polyethylene Wear	3 (1.8%)	0
Osteolysis	3 (1.8%)	0
Recurrent Synovitis	1 (0.6%)	0
Dislocation/Subluxation	2 (1.2%)	0
Survivorship @ 18 yr	98.3%	99.4%

This improvement indicates that the changes made to the LCS to produce the B-P configuration have been effective [118, 120].

6.6.6 The Future

Clinical experience and evaluation of the design concepts and materials currently employed in joint replacement devices will provide information needed to refine or abandon existing designs and to develop new ones. The principal means for design improvement, probably will come from the development of new materials rather than new design concepts.

During the last quarter century, after the development of mobile bearing knees, there has been little improvement is knee joint replacement design. The Oxford knee is basically the same as it was a quarter century ago. The B-P design variants are only slightly improved in that time. Posterior stabilization seems unsound based on engineering principles and clinical experience.

The primary improvements have come from the introduction of ceramic coated titanium alloys and the possible improvement of UHMWPe. Even here the advantages of these materials are somewhat controversial and time is needed to more fully evaluate their benefits.

Probably the greatest impact may come in surgical technique, rather than implant design. The application of computer technology to surgery, although in its infancy, has great potential in producing greatly improved prosthetic alignment, an important, if not critical, need for improved knee joint replacement performance. This is particularly true for mobile bearing unicondylar knee replacement where accurate positioning is more important since all the ligaments are retained. The shape and location of the implants must be such that the functioning of these ligaments is not excessively degraded.

6.7 Conclusion

Analysis, experimentation and clinical results clearly show that two piece, incongruent knees do not provide the stability, mobility and wear resistance of mobile bearing knees. Further, analysis and clinical experience has shown a fundamental flaw in widely used posterior stabilized designs introduced to attempt to solve stability problems with the fixed bearing designs. Only mobile bearing designs have provided needed stability, mobility and long-term wear resistance and survivability that should be expected of well designed implants.

The mobile bearing Mark V B-P Total Knee Replacement is the culmination of more than thirty years of development. It fully exploits the mobile bearing concept by maintaining full congruity in the highly loaded phases of walking motion and fully line contact in the remaining phases and high flexion activities. Further, it provides nearly normal knee motion and stability along with this congruity. The low wear ceramic coating of superior biocompatibility along with its porous coated ingrowth fixation geometry, provide a realistic expectation for a long life and perhaps a lifetime joint replacement.

References

[1]   Nakagawa, S., et al.: Tibial-Femoral Movement 3: Full Flexion in the Living Knee
      Studied by MRI. JBJS 82B(8), 1199–1203 (2000)
[2]   Townsend, M.A., Izak, M., Jackson, R.W.: Total knee motion goniometry. Journal
      of Biomechanics 10, 183–193 (1977)
[3]   Tria, A.J., Klein, K.S., Li, R.-Z.: An Illustrated Guide to the Knee, ch.6. Churchill
      Livingstone, New York (1992)
[4]   Renstrom, P., Johnson, R.L.: Anatomy and biomechanics of the menisci. Clinical
      Sports Medicine 9(3), 523–528 (1990)
[5]   Tria, A.J., Klein, K.S., Li, R.-Z.: An Illustrated Guide to the Knee, ch.2. Churchill
      Livingstone, New York (1992)
[6]   Yoshioka, Y., Cooke, T.D.V.: Geometric Relationships of the Tibia to its
      Mechanical Axis. In: Proceeding of the 32nd Annual ORS, New Orleans, LA,
      p. 384 (1986)
[7]   Morrison, J.B.: The mechanics of the knee joint in relation to normal walking.
      Journal of Biomechanics 3, 51–61 (1970)
[8]   American Academy of Orthopaedic Surgeons, Committee on Biomedical
      Engineering, The patella in TKR - biomedical considerations. Scientific Exhibit,
      59th Annual Meeting of the AAOS (1992)
[9]   Buechel, F.F., et al.: Twenty-year evaluation of meniscal bearing and rotating
      platform knee replacements. Clin. Orthop. 388, 41–50 (2001)
[10] Lennox, D.W., et al.: A histologic comparison of aseptic loosening of cemented,
      press-fit, and biologic ingrowth prostheses. Clinical Orthopaedics 225, 171–191
      (1987)
[11] Rand, J.A., et al.: Kinematic rotating hinge total knee arthroplasty. JBJS 69A, 489–
      497 (1987)
[12] Ivarsson, I., et al.: Long-term follow-up of patients with Geomedic prostheses.
      Archives of Orthopaedic and Traumatic Surgery 105, 353–358 (1986)
[13] Riley, D., et al.: Long -term results of Geomedic total knee replacement. JBJS 66A,
      734 (1984)
[14] Marmor, L.: Unicompartmental arthroplasty of the knee with a minimum ten year
      follow-up period. Clinical Orthopaedics 228, 171 (1988)
[15] Lewallen, D.G., Bryan, R.S., Peterson, L.F.A.: Polycentric total knee arthroplasty:
      A ten year follow-up study. JBJS 66A, 734 (1984)
[16] Nielson, S., et al.: Total condylar knee arthroplasty: A report of 2 - year follow-up
      of 247 cases. Archives of Orthopaedic and Traumatic Surgery 105, 353–358 (1986)
[17] Goldberg, V.M., et al.: Long-term and interim results of the total condylar knee
      arthroplasty   for   osteoarthritis   and   rheumatoid   arthritis.   Orthopaedics
      Transactions 11, 443 (1984)
[18] Sculco, T.P., et al.: Total Condylar III prosthesis in ligament instability.
      Orthopaedic Clinics of North America 20, 221–226 (1989)
[19] Insall, J.N., Lachiewicz, P.F., Burstein, A.H.: The posterior stabilized condylar
      prosthesis: A modification of the total condylar design: Two to four-year clinical
      experience. JBJS 64A, 1317 (1982)
[20] Pappas, M.J., Buechel, F.F.: New Jersey knee simulator. In: Proceedings of the
      Eleventh International Biomaterials Symposium held at Clemson SC, p. 101 (1979)

[21] Mathews, L.S.: Spherocentric arthroplasty of the knee. A long-term and final follow-up evaluation. Clinical Orthopaedics 205, 58–66 (1986)

[22] Insall, J.N., Scott, W.N., Ranawat, C.S.: The Toral Condylar Knee Prosthesis. A Report of Two Hundred and Twenty Cases. JBJS 61A, 173–180 (1979)

[23] Goodfellow, J.W., O'Connor, J.: The mechanics of the knee and prosthesis design. JBJS 60B, 358–367 (1978)

[24] Buechel, F.F., Pappas, M.J.: N.J. Integrated knee replacement system, rationale and review of 193 cases. Biomedical Engineering Corp. Technical Report (1984)

[25] Shindell, R., Neumann, R., Connolly, J.F., Jardon, O.M.: Evaluation of the Noiles hinged knee prosthesis. A five-year study of seventeen knees. JBJS 68A(4), 579–585 (1986)

[26] Buechel, F.F., Pappas, M.J.: New Jersey meniscal bearing knee replacement. U.S. Patent No. 4 340, 978 (1982)

[27] Keblish, A., Pappas, M.J.: Rationale and selection of prosthetic types in mobile bearing total knee arthroplasty. In: AAOS Scientific Exhibit., Presented in Washington, DC (1992)

[28] Hass, B.D., et al.: Kinematic comparison of posterior cruciate sacrifice versus substitution in a mobile bearing total knee arthroplasty. J. Arthroplasty 17, 6 (2002)

[29] Hamelynek, K.J., Stiehl, J.B., Voorhorst, P.: LCS Mobile Bearing Knee Arthroplasty. In: Hamelynek, K.J., Stiehl, J.B. (eds.) LCS Worldwide Multicenter Outcome Study, Section 3. ch.11 (Article 11.2), pp. 212–224. Springer, Heidelberg (2002)

[30] Sorrells, R.B., Stiehl, J.B., Voorhorst, P.E.: Midterm results of mobile-bearing total knee arthroplasty in patients younger than 65 years. Clin. Orthop. 390, 182–189 (2001)

[31] Stiehl, J.B.: The LCS clinical experience - an overview of the literature. In: Hamelynek, K.J., Stiehl, J.B. (eds.) LCS Mobile Bearing Knee Arthroplasty, Section 3. ch.11 (Article 11.1), pp. 209–211. Springer, Heidelberg (2002)

[32] Stiehl, J.B.: Frontal plane kinematics after mobile bearing total knee arthroplasty. Clin. Orthop. 392, 56–61 (2001)

[33] Pappas, M.J.: Mobile Bearing Total Joint Replacement. U.S. Patent No. 5, 683, 468 (1997)

[34] Index Total Knee System, http://orthosupersite.com/view.asp?rID=40642

[35] Gupta, S.K., Ranawat, A.S., Shah, V., Zikria, B.A., Zikria, J.F., Ranawat, C.S.: The P.F.C. sigma RP-F TKA designed for improved performance: a matched-pair study. Orthop. 29(9 suppl.), S49–S52 (2006)

[36] Multiple mobile bearing knee designs are now available. Orthopaedics Today – International Edition, 1 (July/August 1998)

[37] Morgan-Jones, R., Roger, G., Solis, G., Parish, E., Cross, M.: Meniscal bearing uncemented total knee arthroplasty. The Journal of Arthroplasty 18(1), 41–44 (1998)

[38] Schai, P.A., Thornhill, T.S., Scott, R.D.: Total knee arthroplasty with the PFC system; Relults at aminimum of ten years survivorship analysis. JBJS 80B(5), 850–958 (1998)

[39] Jones, S.M.G., et al.: Polyethylene wear in uncemented knee replacements. JBJS 74B, 18–22 (1992)

[40] Colizza, W.A., Insall, J.N., Scuderi, G.R.: The posterior stabilized total knee prosthesis. Assessment of polyethylene damage and osteolysis after a ten-year minimum follow-up. JBJS 77(65), 619 (1995)

[41] Ritter, M.A., Campbell, E., Farix, P.M., et al.: Long-term survival analysis of the posterior cruciate condylar total knee arthroplasty. A 10-year evaluation. J. Arthroplasty 4, 293 (1989)

[42] Font-Rodriguez, D.E., Scuderi, G.R., Insall, J.N.: Survivorship of cemented total knee arthroplasty. Clin. Orthop. Relat. Res. 79 (1997)

[43] Lachiewicz, P.F., Soileau, E.S.: The rates of osteolysis and; loosening associated with s modular posterior stabilized knee replacement- - Results at five to fourteen years. JBJS 86A(3), 525–530 (2004)

[44] Bolanos, A.A., et al.: A comparison of isokinetic strength testing and gait analysis in patients with posterior cruciate-retaining and substituting knee Arthroplasties. J. Arthroplasty 13(8) (1998)

[45] Kocmond, J.H., Delp, S.L., Stern, S.: Stability and range of motion of Insall-Burstein condylar prosthesis. J. Arthroplasty 10(3) (1995)

[46] Lombardi, A.V., et al.: Late versus early engagement of posterior stabilized prostheses: effect on extensor moment arm and resultant extensor loads. In: 68th Annual Meeting on AAOS Scientific Exhibit SE023, San Francisco, CA (February 2001)

[47] Banks, S.A., Harmon, M.K., Hodge, W.A.: Mechanism of anterior impingement damage in total knee arthroplasty. J. JBJS 84A (2001)

[48] Mariconda, M., Lotti, G., Milano, C.: Fracture of posterior-stabilized tibial insert in genesis knee prosthesis. J. Arthroplasty 15(4) (2000)

[49] Mestha, P., Shenava, Y., D'Arcy, J.C.: Fracture of the polyethylene tibial post in posterior stabilized (Insall Burstein II) total knee arthroplasty. J. Arthroplasty 15, 814–815 (2000)

[50] Bal, B.S., Greenberg, D., Li, S., et al.: Tibial post failures in a condylar posterior cruciate substituting total knee arthroplasty. J. Arthroplasty 23(5) (2008)

[51] Clarke, H.D., Math, K.R., Scuderi, G.R.: Polyethylene post failure in posterior stabilized total knee arthroplasty. J. Arthroplasty 19, 529 (2004)

[52] Puloski, S.K., McCalden, R.W., MacDonald, S.J., et al.: Tibial post wear in posterior stabilized total knee arthroplasty. An unrecognized source of polyethylene debris. JBJS 83A, 390 (2001)

[53] Chiu, Y.S., Chen, W.M., Huang, C.K., et al.: Fracture of the polyethylene tibial post in a NexGen PS posterior stabilized knee prosthesis. J. Arthroplasty 19, 1045 (2004)

[54] Callaghan, J.J., et al.: Tibial post impingement in posterior-stabilized total knee arthroplasty. Clin. Orthop. Relat. Res. 404, 83–88 (2002)

[55] Furman, B.D., Lipman, J., Kligman, M., et al.: Tibial post wear in posterior-stabilized knee replacements is design dependent. Clin. Orthop. Related Res. 466(11), 2650–2655 (2008)

[56] Akasagi, Y., Matsuda, S., Shimoto, T., et al.: Contact stress analysis of the conforming post-cam mechanism in posterior-stabilized total knee arthroplasty. J. Arthroplasty 23, 736 (2008)

[57] Morra, E.A., Greewald, A.S.: Polymer insert stress in total knee designs during high-flexion activities: A finite element study. JBJS 87A, 120–124 (2005)

[58] Anderson, M.J., Becker, D.L., Kieckbusch, T.: Patellofemoral complications after stabilized total knee arthroplasty. J. Arthroplasty 17(4) (2002)

[59] Beight, J.L., et al.: The "patellar, clunk" syndrome after stabilized total knee arthroplasty. Clin. Orthop. 299, 139–142 (1994)

[60] Hozack, W.J., et al.: The patellar clunk syndrome -a complication of posterior-stabilized total knee arthroplasty. Clin. Orthop. 241, 203–208 (1989)

[61] Tria Jr., A.L., et al.: Patellar fractures in posterior stabilized knee Arthroplasties. Clin. Orthop. 299, 131–138 (1994)

[62] Rapp, S.M.: Patellar crepitus: A nagging but treatable problem related to posterior-stabilized TKR. Orthosipersite (2009)

[63] Lombardi, A.V., et al.: Intercondylar distal femoral fracture –an unreported complication of posterior-stabilized total knee arthroplasty. J. Arthroplasty 10(5) (1995)

[64] Pollock, D.C., Ammeen, D., Engh, G.A.: Synovial entrapment: a complication of posterior stabilized total knee arthroplasty. JBJS 84A, 2174–2178 (2002)

[65] Mikulak, S.A., et al.: Loosening and osteolysis with the press-fit condylar posterior-cruciate-substituting total knee replacement. JBJS 83A, 398–403 (2001)

[66] Choi, W.C., Lee, S., Seong, S.C., et al.: Comparison Between Standard and High-Flexion Posterior-Stabilized Rotating-Platform Mobile-Bearing Total Knee Arthoplasties: A Randomized Controlled Study. JBJS (A) 92-A, 2634–2642 (2010)

[67] Ranawat, A.S., Blum, Y., Maheshwari, A., et al.: Matched pair comparison of rotating platform and fixed bearing knees; 5year follow-up. Presented at ASTM Symposium on Mobile Bearing Total Knee Replacement Devices, St. Louis, MO (May 18, 2010)

[68] Fukunag, K., Kobayashi, A., Minoda, Y., et al.: The incidence of patellar clunk syndrome in a recently designed mobile-bearing posteriorly stabilized total knee replacement. JBJS (Br) 91-B, 463–468 (2009)

[69] Morra, E.A., Greenwald, A.S.: Polymer Insert Stress in Total Knee Designs During High-Flexion Activities: A Finite Element Study. JBJS (A) 87-A(suppl. 2), 120–124 (2005)

[70] Kim, Y.H., Kim, J.-S.: Comparison of Anterior-Posterior-Glide and Rotating-Platform Low Contact Stress Mobile-Bearing Total Knee Arthroplasties. JBJS 86, 1239–1247 (2004)

[71] Bartel, D.L., Bicknell, V.U., Wright, T.M.: The effect of conformity, thickness and material on stresses in ultra-high molecular weight polyethylene components for total joint replacement. JBJS 68A, 1041–1053 (1986)

[72] Matauda, S., Whiteside, L.A., White, S.E.: The effect of varus tilt on contact stresses in total knee arthroplasty: a biomechanical study. Orthopaedics 22(3), 303–307 (1999)

[73] Pappas, M.J., Makris, G., Buechel, F.F.: Evaluation of contact stresses in metal-plastic total knee replacements. In: Pizzoferrato, A. (ed.) Biomaterials and Clinical Applications, pp. 259–264. Elsevier Science Publishers B.V, Amsterdam (1987)

[74] Dorr, L.D., Ochsner, J.L., Gronley, J., et al.: Functional comparison of posterior cruciate-retaining vs. sacrificing TKA. Clin. Orthop. 236, 36–43 (1988)

[75] Hamelynek, K.J., Stiehl, J.B., Voorhorst, P.: LCS Mobile Bearing Knee Arthroplasty. In: Hamelynek, K.J., Stiehl, J.B. (eds.) LCS Worldwide Multicenter Outcome Study. Springer, Heidelberg (2002)

[76] Sorrells, R.B., Stiehl, J.B., Voorhorst, P.E.: Midterm results of mobile-bearing total knee arthroplasty in patients younger than 65 years. Clin. Orthop. 390, 182–189 (2001)

[77] Stiehl, J.B.: The LCS clinical experience - an overview of the literature. In: Hamelynek, K.J., Stiehl, J.B. (eds.) LCS Mobile Bearing Knee Arthroplasty. Springer, Heidelberg (2002)

[78] Ranawat, A.S., Gupta, S.K., Ranawat, C.S.: The P.F.C. sigma RP-F total knee arthroplasty: designed for improved performance. Orthop. 29(9 Suppl.), S28–S29 (2006)

[79] Stiehl, J.B., et al.: Frontal plane kinematics after mobile bearing total knee arthroplasty. Clin. Orthop. 392, 56–61 (2001)

[80] Nagura, T., Dyrby, C.O., Alexander, E.J., et al.: Mechanical loads at the knee joint during deep flexion. J. Orthro. Res. 4, 881 (2002)

[81] Walker, P.S.: Human Joints and Their Artificial Replacements. Charles Thomas, Springfield, Illinois (1978)

[82] Deutschman, A.D., Michels, W.J., Wilson, C.E.: Factor of Safety. Machine Design-Theory and Practice. Section 1-1, 8-11 and Section 10-16. Macmillan Publishing Co., New York (1975)

[83] Sealy, F.B., Smith, J.O.: Advanced Mechanics of Materials. Wiley and Sons, New York (1958)

[84] Hostalen, G.U.R.: Hoechst Aktiengesellschaft, Verkauf Kunstoffe. 6230 Frankfurt am Main 80, 22 (1982)

[85] Lombardi, A.V., et al.: Dislocation following primary posterior stabilized total knee arthroplasty. J. Arthroplasty 8, 6 (1993)

[86] Ochsner Jr., U., Kostman, W.C., Dodson, M.: Posterior dislocation of a posterior-stabilized total knee arthroplasty -a report of two Cases. Am. J. Orthop., 310–312 (1996)

[87] Hamai, S., Muira, H., Higaki, H., et al.: Evaluation of impingement of the anterior tibial post during gait in a posterior-stabilized total knee replacement. JBJ 90B(8), 1180–1185 (2000)

[88] Li, G., Papannagari, R., Most, E., et al.: Anterior post impingement in a posterior stabilized total knee arthroplasty. J. Orthop. Res. 23, 536–541 (2005)

[89] McEwan, H.M.J., et al.: Wear of fixed bearing and rotating platform mobile bearing knees subject to high levels of internal and external axial rotation. J. of Material Science: Materials in Medicine 12, 1049–1052 (2001)

[90] Buechel, F.F.: B-P Tricompartmental Knee – Surgical Procedure. Brochure C-019m, Biomedical Engineering Trust, Naples FL (2008)

[91] Argenson, J.N., O'Connor, J.: Polyethylene wear in meniscal knee replacement: A one to nine year retrieval analysis. JBJS 74B, 228–232 (1992)

[92] Barrett, D.S., et al.: The Oxford knee replacement: a review from an independent centre. JBJS 72B, 775–778 (1990)

[93] Carr, A.J., Keyes, G., Miller, R.K.: Medial unicompartmental arthroplasty: A survival study of the Oxford meniscal bearing knee. Presented at the Ninth Combined Meeting of the Orthopaedic Association of the English Speaking World (Poster Exhibit), held at Toronto Canada, June 21-26 (1992)

[94] Pappas, M.J., Buechel, F.F.: On The Use Of A Constant Radius Femoral Component in Meniscal Bearing Knee Replacement. J. of Orthopaedic Rheumatology 7, 27–29 (1994)

[95] Pappas, M.J., Makris, G., Buechel, F.F.: Contact stresses in metal-plastic total knee replacements: A theoretical and experimental study. Biomedical Engineering Technical Report (1986)

[96]   McNamara, J.L., Collier, J.P., Mayor, M.B.: Sensitivity of Current Total Knee Prosthesis to Tibiofemoral Malalignment Poster Exhibit A24. In: 61st Annual Meeting of the AAOS at New Orleans, LA (1994)

[97]   White, J.E., Selby, J.: The effect of loading and flexion on area contact in the knee. In: Transactions of the 39th Meeting of the ORS, San Francisco CA, p. 423 (1993)

[98]   Buechel, F.F., Pappas, M.J., Makris, G.: Evaluation of contact stress in metal backed patellar replacements; A predictor of survivorship. Clinical Orthopeadics and Related Research 273, 190–197 (1991)

[99]   Stulberg, S.D., et al.: Failure mechanisms of metal-backed patellar components. Clinical Orthopaedics and Related Research 236, 88–105 (1988)

[100]   Bourne, R.B., et al.: Metal-backed total knee replacement patellar components: a major problem for the future. Presented at the 58th Annual Meeting of the AAOS (1990)

[101]   Lewallen, D.G., Rand, J.R.: Failure of metal-backed patellar components following total knee replacement. Presented at the 58th Annual Meeting of the AAOS (1990)

[102]   Collier, J.P., et al.: Examination of porous-coated patellar components and analysis of the reasons for their retrieval. Presented at the 58th Annual Meeting of the AAOS (1990)

[103]   Tokgozoglu, A.M., et al.: Patellar complications in total knee arthroplasty. Presented at the 58th Annual Meeting of the AAOS (1990)

[104]   Wasilewski, S.A., et al.: Patellofemoral complications after total knee arthroplasty. Presented at the 58th Annual Meeting of the AAOS (1990)

[105]   Chess, D.G., et al.: Patellofemoral complications with the Miller-Galante total knee. Presented at the 58th Annual Meeting of the AAOS (1990)

[106]   Pappas, M.J., Makris, G., Buechel, F.F.: Wear in prosthetic knee joints. In: Scientific Exhibit, 59th Annual Meeting of the AAOS, Washington, DC (1992)

[107]   Postac, P.D., Matejczyk, M.-B., Greenwald, A.S.: Stability characteristics of total knee replacements. In: Scientific Exhibit, 56th Annual Meeting of the AAOS (1989)

[108]   Buechel, F.F., Pappas, M.J.: Long-term survivorship analysis of cruciate-sparing vs. cruciate sacrificing knee prostheses using meniscal bearings. Clinical Orthopaedics 260, 162–169 (1990)

[109]   Sorrells, R.B., et al.: Clinical results and survivorship of cemented and uncemented cruciate sacrificing total knee replacements. In: Scientific Exhibit, 59th Meeting of the AAOS (1991)

[110]   Collier, J.: Personal communication (1994)

[111]   Morra, E.A., Greewald, A.S.: Polymer insert stress in total knee designs during high-flexion activities: A finite element study. JBJS 87A, 120–124 (2005)

[112]   Chin, K.R., et al.: Intraoperative measurements of male and female distal femurs during primary total knee Arthroplasty. J. Knee Surg. 15(4), 213–217 (2002) ISSN: 1538-8506

[113]   Dupont, C.G.: Comparison of three standard radiologic techniques for screening of patellar subluxations. Clinics in Sports Medicine 21(3), 389–401 (2000)

[114]   Conditt, M.A., et al.: Backside Wear of Polyethylene Tibial Inserts: Machanisim and Magnitude of Material Loss. JBJS 87A(2), 326–331 (2005)

[115]   Mensch, J.S., Amstutz, H.C.: Knee morphology as a guide to knee replacement. Clinical Orthopaedics and Related Research 112, 235–241 (1975)

[116] Keblish, P.A., Greenwald, A.S.: Comparison of patella retention and patella replacement in LCS mobile bearing total knee arthroplasty: A prospective comparison of 52 knees in 26 patients. Presented at the 58th Annual meeting of the AAOS (1990)

[117] Mockford, B.J., Beverland, D.R.: Secondary Resurfacing of the Patella in Mobile Bearing Total Knee Arthroplasty. The Journal of Arthroplasty 20(7), 901–988 (2005)

[118] Buechel, F.F., et al.: 31year evolution of the rotatiing platfoerm TKR: coping with "spinout" and wear. Presented at the ASTM International nSymposium on Mobile Bearing Devices, St. Lousi MO (2010) (in press)

[119] Pappas, M.J., et al.: Comparison of Wear Of UHMWPe Cups Articulating With CoCr and TiN Coated Femoral Heads. Transactions of the Society of Biomaterials XIII, 36 (1990)

[120] Buechel Sr., F.F., et al.: Sr et al Twenty-year evaluation of the New Jaresy LCS rotating platform knee replacement. K. Knee Surg. 15, 84–89 (2002)